CORONA CITY

Voices from an Epicenter

Praise for
Corona City: Voices from an Epicenter

Corona City is a collection of compelling, intimate stories that reveal the resilience of New Jerseyans and New Yorkers amid the losses, fears, and uncertainties of the historic COVID-19 pandemic outbreak. This book gives a glimpse into the high cost of an all-too-real pandemic affecting individual lives, minds, and hearts. I have been a proud resident of New Jersey or New York nearly all my life, and I grieve the toll this virus has taken on two states I love. I applaud *Corona City* for bringing us these stories.

— Christine Todd Whitman
Former New Jersey governor and EPA administrator
Author, *It's My Party Too: The Battle for the Heart of the GOP* and the *Future of America*
(Penguin Books, 2005)

The writers and photographers of *Corona City* offer readers vivid recollections of devastation and survival from the virus's peak. Together, we mourn and celebrate in this tangible history for future generations. Read this book to remember and find the hope within yourself and our collective human story.

— Chloe Yelena Miller
Author, *Viable* (Lily Poetry Review Books, 2021)

Through their personal experiences, the contributors to *Corona City* document what life is like under the pall of COVID-19. Everything is here—literally from birth to death, from extraordinary acts of front-line response to coping with the loneliness of quarantine. Despite the urgency of the words and images, this book feels timeless as these writers and photographers offer glimpses of hope amid the wreckage. This is a heartbreaking, necessary, and moving act of witness.

— Sue William Silverman
Author, *How to Survive Death and Other Inconveniences*
(University of Nebraska Press, 2020)

As a COVID-19 survivor and psychologist who lives and works in New York City, I find this phenomenal and timely book to be both validating and healing. It captures the fears, challenges, and triumphs of our metropolis during this pandemic through shared stories and intimate photos, and it gives voice to all that we continue to struggle with. *Corona City* reminds us that despite our losses, we are resilient and will come together in community and not only survive but eventually thrive.

— Dr. Heidi Horsley

Executive director, Open to Hope Foundation; Adjunct professor, Columbia University
Author, *Open to Hope: Inspirational Stories for Handling the Holidays after Loss*
(Open to Hope Foundation, 2011)

This extraordinary book allows the reader to enter the hell realm that New York and New Jersey became in spring 2020—a hell realm populated by extraordinary, selfless angels. The COVID-19 pandemic has revealed vulnerabilities and weaknesses in our nation. But it has also revealed the ever-present magnificence of the human spirit. With exquisite, powerful writing, *Corona City* reveals the true, on-the-ground scope of this turning point in human history. It also presents signposts that point the way to where humanity can and must go—if we and our planet are to survive.

— John E. Welshons

Author, *When Prayers Aren't Answered* (New World Library, 2010)

Illuminating firsthand accounts, beautifully written and closely observed, that add up to the panoramic big picture.

— Dar Williams

Singer-songwriter
Author, *What I Found in a Thousand Towns* (Basic Books, 2017)]

CORONA CITY

Voices from an Epicenter

Edited by Lorraine Ash

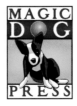

MAGIC DOG PRESS

Corona City: Voices from an Epicenter

Cover Photo: *Rush Hour*
A nearly vacant Main Concourse of Grand Central Station
during what normally is a bustling afternoon rush hour, March 30, 2020
(Photo by Matthijs Noome)

Published by Magic Dog Press, LLC
PO Box 108
Milton Freewater, OR 97862
For information contact Sherry Wachter, sherry@sherrywachter.com

Library of Congress Cataloging-in-Publishing Data

Ash, Lorraine, Editor
Corona City: Voices from an Epicenter

p. cm.

ISBN 978-1-7357245-0-8

Pandemic—Covid-19—Corona Virus   2.Covid-19—Personal Stories 3. Covid-19—Impacts 4. Corona Virus—United States

RC 150.4 139 2020   362.9162 Co

10 9 8 7 6 5 4 3 2 1

DEDICATED TO
COVID-19 VICTIMS
WORLDWIDE

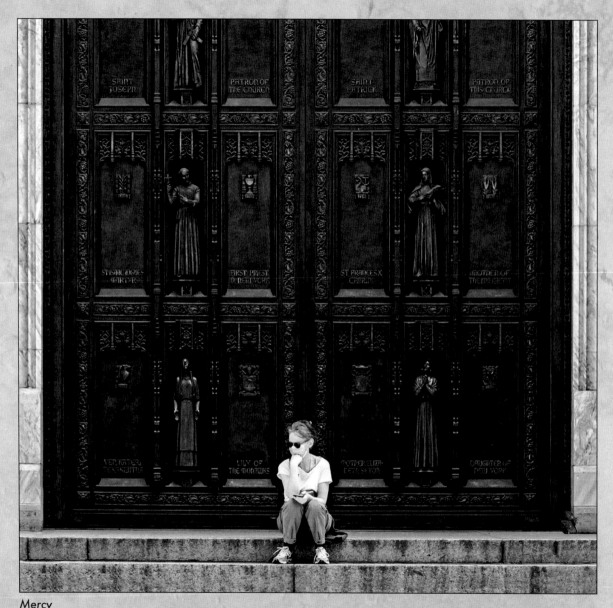

Mercy
A woman sits in front of a closed Saint Patrick's Cathedral during New York City's COVID-19 lockdown, May 22, 2020
(Photo by Jessica Margo)

Contents

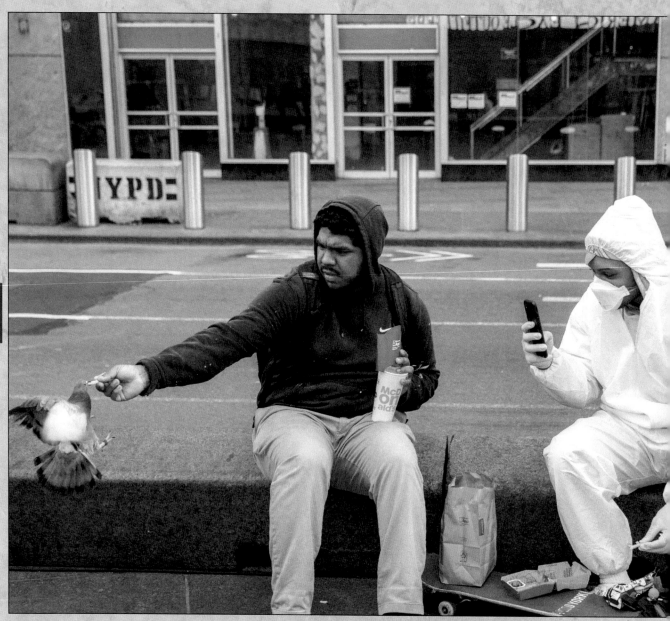

Meal Time
Times Square, March 24, 2020 (Photo by Walter Wlodarczyk)

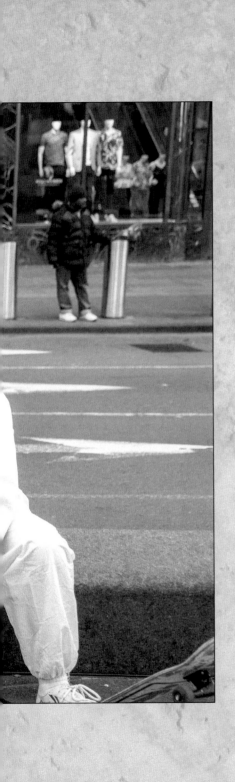

Introduction

Fear and uncertainty permeated the very air we breathed in New York and New Jersey in early March 2020.

Neighbors and loved ones grew suddenly, seriously ill. COVID-19 patients overflowed our hospitals. Ambulances zoomed along city streets, sirens wailing. The stock market crashed. Workplaces closed. Broadway went dark. Shoppers hoarded toilet paper and paper towels, meats and chicken, even garlic, leaving some supermarket shelves empty.

Simultaneously, conflicting reports jammed our news circuits: Don't wear a mask, they stated, but wear gloves. If you touch surfaces, sanitize your hands. Sanitize your groceries. Sanitize your mail. Then the mandate to wear masks arrived.

Amid it all, we were alone in our homes—locked down.

Meanwhile, the Center at Mariandale, a retreat house that sits majestically along the Hudson River, closed its physical doors. The campus, sponsored by the Dominican Sisters of Hope, is in Westchester County, New York, close to the epicenter ravaged by the coronavirus in those early days.

In the spirit of the sisters' mission, Mariandale wanted to provide services for a panicked, terrified public. It wanted to create community. There was only one place to bring people together—online. Mariandale did so with the help of Jane Hanley, its administrator, and Karen Bernard, its program coordinator. They very quickly began offering new programming on Zoom. It had to be free. After all, income everywhere was wiped out.

The Catholic call to service felt familiar. I'd grown up with it. So I created *COVID-19 Diaries: Writing in the Age of Pandemic.* I designed this four-week workshop as a place people could share experiences and bear witness wherever they were—on breadlines, front lines, or unemployment lines, in sickbeds, or at home, anywhere.

Thirty-five people joined us. They wrote stories, straight from their lives and hearts, free of political agendas or any preconceived notions. Their words held power. Clearly, an intimate history of the pandemic was emerging. Collectively, their voices formed a mosaic of how life really was in the age of the coronavirus— what it sounded like, smelled like, felt like.

Mid-series, I joined forces with one of the participants, Sherry Wachter of Magic Dog Press. We both envisioned *Corona City,* an anthology of these voices.

But the project needed even more viewpoints. Adhering to the six degrees of separation idea, I invited the Mariandale writers to draw in others in their sphere. I did likewise, even holding a second *COVID-19 Diaries* Zoom forum.

The sixty-one writers whose work is included in this book (and an online gallery supplementing the book) include COVID survivors and those of us who, like me, lost someone they knew to the virus. Among the others are nurses, bestselling memoirists, two owners of small businesses deemed "nonessential," teachers, a doctor, mask makers, a laid-off news photographer, an EMT captain, an opera singer, a nutritionist in a nursing home, gardeners, a pianist, an addiction counselor, a mother of three, a cancer patient, and a Corona Courier, one in the army of citizen cyclists who made free, safe, contactless deliveries throughout New York City to anyone who needed groceries and other supplies.

A call for photography during the lockdown yielded twenty stunning portfolios of images taken from the Bronx down to the Jersey Shore.

At a certain point I realized we'd fulfilled the Mariandale vision: People had come together and written about their extraordinary experiences and states of mind. They'd created community now and a record for the historians of tomorrow. It was time to publish.

You, the readers, complete the experience and the mission when you buy and read a copy of this anthology.

One hundred percent of *Corona City* sales benefits Feeding America, a nationwide network of more than two hundred food banks that feed millions of Americans through food pantries, shelters, soup kitchens, and other community initiatives. The nonprofit points to a solitary, staggering statistic: more than 54 million Americans may go hungry in 2020 because of the coronavirus.

That means hunger threatens Americans' well-being and survival as much as the virus itself. In this important respect America is not great. It is greatly, historically, massively weakened. All of us are diminished when any of us lack life's basic necessities.

As this unbridled American tragedy continues, we in the New York Metro Area realize the whole country is now "Corona City." We feel for the suffering and death in the new epicenters and the healthcare workers who imperil themselves to treat patients, some of them victims of their own behavior.

And we realize the virus isn't done with any of us yet. We could see another wave here in the Mid-Atlantic states. At least our citizens seem to think so. People are already stockpiling paper products, sanitizers, and masks in advance.

Thank you for caring enough to read us. Keep reading. Keep holding honest, informed conversations. Keep adding to the collective conscience that will remember what we are enduring. And never for a moment, especially now, doubt the power of a camera, a pen, or the people.

Lorraine Ash

ALLENDALE, NJ
AUGUST 2020

ARRIVAL

COVID-19 took us by surprise though it shouldn't have. There were reports and rumblings about it for months. We heard mixed messages, though, including presidential reassurances that it would disappear "like a miracle," weaken in the spring warmth, and that 99 percent of cases are "totally harmless." We even heard the coronavirus was a hoax. But the real story set in when our friends and loved ones were struck down.

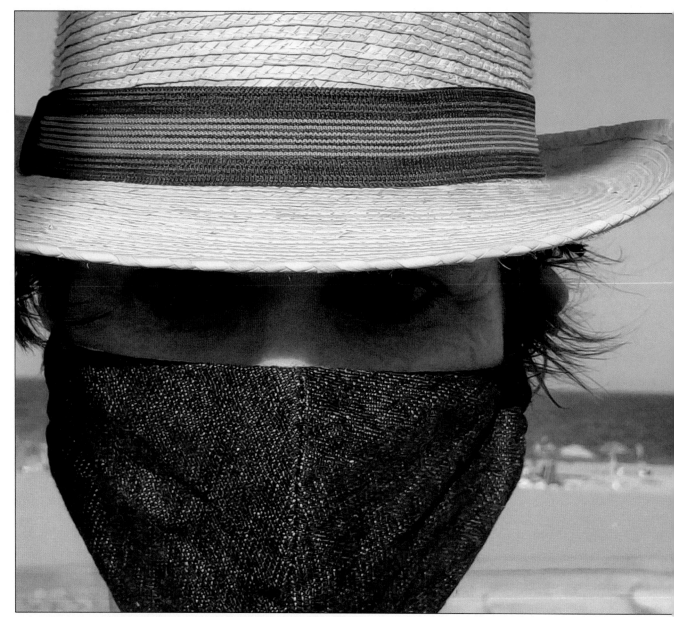

Jen Singer, masked and socially distant, at Sea Bright Public Beach in
Sea Bright, New Jersey, during the summer of 2020 (Photo by Jen Singer)

COVID-19 Broke My Heart

Jen Singer

Even though my new pacemaker's instructions didn't specifically say, "Don't jump off lifeguard stands," I knew enough to climb back down. Two months after COVID-19 left me with a third-degree heart block and heart failure, I recognized that even the fleeting idea of making a flying dismount from six feet above the sand was a tiny victory. It meant that I was feeling better. Also, that I might need adult supervision.

I'd come to the beach near my house at the Jersey Shore because I knew nobody was there. The Weather Channel's radar showed that the thunderstorms we'd had all afternoon were blowing out to sea, and the Sea Bright Live Surf Cam revealed a gloriously empty public beach. So I packed up my face mask, the homemade one with red, white, and blue sailboats, and drove to the beach, sunroof open, blasting E Street Radio.

I almost felt normal. Almost. I'm not sure I'll ever feel normal again.

I caught COVID in February, either on a train to Boston or a plane to Seattle. I am sure I spread it to other people, but hardly anyone was testing for coronavirus in the US on February 24, let alone an urgent care center in rural Washington State, where I'd gone to work on my memoir. The doctor ruled out pneumonia, influenza A and B, and strep throat. I spent a few extra days out west trying to get healthy enough to fly back home.

Looking back, I realize I had classic COVID symptoms: cough, fever, and nausea. I even threw up. But it felt like a mild bronchitis, and within a few weeks, I was all better. Or so I thought.

I made a pandemic purchase that would set off a series of health problems that eventually landed me in the ER, surrounded by healthcare professionals in Personal Protective Equipment (PPE). I'd bought one of those tennis rebounders I'd seen in my Instagram feed. I was hitting the ball, which was fastened to a very long rubber rope, in my backyard when I ran out of steam. Gasping for air, I thought, *Gee, I must still have that virus.* So I put away my tennis racquet and took it easy.

Two days later, I started getting shortness of breath and dizziness when walking upstairs. My house has three flights of stairs. That Friday in early April, an urgent care doctor encouraged me to come in for a COVID test, presumably because I'd said the magic words: "travel," "Seattle," and "son returned home from New York City." It would be a week before I got the results.

By Monday, my abdomen felt as though there wasn't enough room for my organs, like when you're eight months pregnant and the baby squashes everything in there. I called the urgent care doctor, who told me to go to the hospital because she thought I might be having a gallstone attack. I didn't want to go, because there was COVID at the hospital, and what if I caught it? But I knew I needed to go.

On the back of an envelope I wrote out the passwords to my computer and my bank and credit card accounts, phone numbers for relatives and family friends, and contact information for my doctors and my health insurance company. I handed it to my son, Nick, a senior in college whose campus had shut down two weeks earlier. He drove me to the ER. I went in alone.

Lucky for me, I'd spent a lot of time in hospitals when I had lymphoma in 2007, so I was adept at unplugging all my wires and tubes to various monitors and such. When the ER nurses were too busy, which was every time, I could take myself to the bathroom. Unfortunately, though, lymphoma—or the treatments for it—would be the reason I wound up in the ER in the first place.

From my gurney in the pediatric ER room (it was the only free room), I watched three healthcare workers watch my EKG results on the monitor behind me.

"First degree block … no, second," the doctor said from behind her mask and face shield.

"Wait, third?" a nurse offered.

"Yes, third," the doctor confirmed. It meant I had a life-threatening condition: the electrical system of my heart had stopped doing its job.

And that's how I wound up with a pacemaker at age fifty-three. A tennis-playing, Sedona-hiking, gym-going fifty-three. My cardiologist—now I have a cardiologist—surmised that chemo and radiation had damaged my heart and that COVID had found it and sped up the process, or something like that. Without COVID I may have made it well into old age before my heart gave out, or at least until Medicare foots the hospital bill. Now I'm not so sure about my odds of being around long enough to get Medicare.

I spent two days on the COVID floor before a rapid test came up negative and they moved me to Cardiology. On the first night, a nurse found me returning from the bathroom, wires in my hand, and asked how I was feeling.

"My chest hurts a little," I said.

Okay, so never say "my chest hurts a little" on the Cardiology floor. Moments later, I was surrounded by a team of medical experts led by a concerned cardiologist, much like I suppose SEAL Team Six works.

"Aha," I said, assuring them I was not in cardiac arrest. "I'm used to Oncology where you report your pain levels." Note to self: *don't say 'pain' on this floor unless it's a cardiac emergency.*

The night before my pacemaker surgery, nurses watched my heart rate on the monitors at their station all night. When it dropped to thirty-eight, they worried they might have to "paddle" me with a defibrillator. My ejection fraction, the rate at which the heart pumps blood to the organs, was just 40 percent—heart failure, though the nonischemic kind, which means my arteries are as clear as the Lincoln Tunnel during the lockdown.

The day after my pacemaker surgery, the urgent care doctor called me with the results of my first COVID test—positive. I'd been on the Cardiology floor, maskless, for three days. I rang the nurse and asked for a nurse to come to my room. I didn't want to announce, "I have COVID," over the intercom. When no one came, I rang again.

"Um, I just found out I'm positive for COVID."

I was quickly wheeled back over to the COVID floor where things had changed. All of the doors to the rooms were closed, and the nurses crowded the hallway in full PPE, like the Ghostbusters waiting for a call. My room had a common household fan in the window that was blowing in 45-degree air from off the river, which was engulfed in whitecaps. The heater was on full blast, but it was no match. I put on my parka and waited five hours for my discharge papers before I could finally go home to a two-week quarantine. Nick made my meals and left them at my bedroom door.

The day I drove to the beach, my ejection fraction was still just 40 percent, a disappointing post-hospital finding that means my pacemaker isn't helping to boost my heart's output. But I started taking new medication designed to improve symptoms so that I'm less out of breath on stairs and more likely to consider jumping off lifeguard stands. The hope is to get my ejection fraction up toward normal—50 percent. If it doesn't, I'll have to adjust to a "new normal," and if cancer taught me anything, it's that there's nothing normal about "new normal."

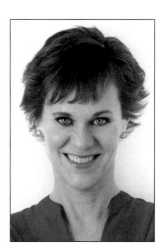

Jen Singer is a writer and writing coach in Red Bank, New Jersey. She is a Non-Hodgkin's lymphoma and COVID-19 survivor with a season beach badge that's gathering dust during the pandemic.

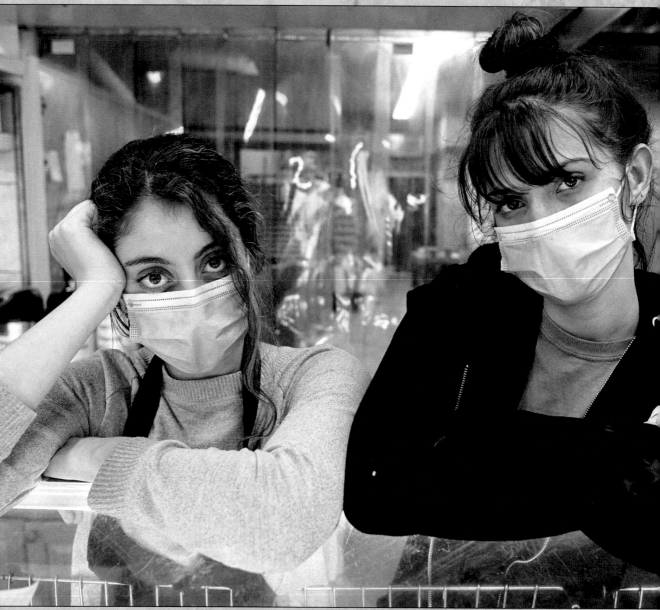

Bagels and Lockdown
Workers at The Bagel Shoppe in Hackensack, New Jersey take a break to
pose for a photo on April 29, 2020 (Photo by Christopher Monroe)

The Intrusion

Jan Keyes

February–March 2020

The news blared out a quirky story. A cruise ship's passengers were quarantined because of an unknown virus. I sneered at the huge ocean liner spanning the TV screen. People were lounging on their luxurious floating hotel balconies. *So what? They had their fun. They'll just have to endure another week of vacation. Who cares?*

Within the week death statistics were tacked onto the follow-up stories. New words were repeated daily: "epidemic" turned into "worldwide pandemic." *Worldwide? Uncontrollable? Deadly? Hardly. So a couple of cases leaked into Washington State. No big deal.*

Then daily updates turned into dire warnings that turned into legal restrictions. *They want us to be quarantined? What's going on?*

When I first donned a face mask and walked into a store, I felt my hot breath under my nose. *This is strange. Everyone's going to stare at me.* No one did. People walked around like zombies, learning to keep an arm's length from each other. Taped markings on the floor reminded me to pay attention, to watch others—not a concept I was used to. City life early on had taught me the opposite: don't pay attention and don't draw attention from strangers. I found myself monitoring my sacred invisible space for any infractions. As I tried to escape the canned goods aisle, a lady concentrating on brand comparisons backed into my shopping cart. *Geez! I need more than a mask, I need full body armor!*

"Oh, I'm sorry," she said, as she slid back to her cart. I grunted. *Why can't she watch what she's doing?*

By late February the pandemic was on everyone's mind, even infecting conversations. At my temp office job everyone was leery of getting too close. Our sentences became stilted, as if the very words spoken through masks could do harm. An occasional cough brought glares and put all of us on edge.

"It's just a dry throat. Allergies, you know," someone in the back explained.

I loosened my tightened fists and closed lips behind my mask and sensed everyone else did, too. We all circumvented the masked cougher, at least for the next few minutes.

By early March my job of warmly greeting customers, offering a cup of coffee, and chatting turned into a solemn affair. Even if I could offer a smile, it couldn't be seen. Customers were required to remain outside, even on wintry days. Papers, exchanged with latex-gloved hands, were passed through locked doors. I apologized every time. There was nothing I could do.

A woman seated outside was filling out requisite forms. I saw her shivering, retrieved my cape, and quickly threw it around her shoulders. She looked up at me gratefully.

"Thank you. I didn't know what to expect," she said.

"Nobody does," I replied before returning to safety behind the glass doors.

When she left and handed me my cape, my coworkers chided me.

"You shouldn't have done that," one said. "That's not a good idea."

I pinched the cape in my outstretched fingers and tossed it on a nearby chair, as if I'd just stepped out of a leper colony.

Customers wanted to quicken their transactions, even avoiding eye contact. When our gazes met, we each silently narrowed our focus, acknowledging our unsaid fears. *Could this one have it? Could this one betray my health and transmit the invisible contagion?*

Sometimes customers phoned to let me know they'd drop off their work. When they arrived, I went outside to meet them. Their parked car still running, they barely rolled down their window enough to slide their envelope into my hands.

"Okay, thanks," I said, my voice muffled through my mask as they sped away.

Cordiality had taken on a threatening new meaning. Silence was safer.

In between customers I wiped down my pens with a slurry of sanitizers and sprayed the credit card machine and keyboard to ease my pent-up anxieties. *Could I be holding the virus in my hand, squeezed under my thumb in this new batch of papers?* I stared down. *This all seems like a weird dream.* I said as much to one coworker. She nodded in silence.

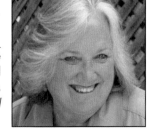

Jan Keyes, born in Chicago, now lives in bucolic Warren County, New Jersey where she enjoys gardening, practicing herbalism, tending to her two cats, the wildlife, and being with Joe, her loving husband of more than thirty years. A published author, she is currently working on her forthcoming memoir, *Ward of the State: Surviving Childhood Without Family.*

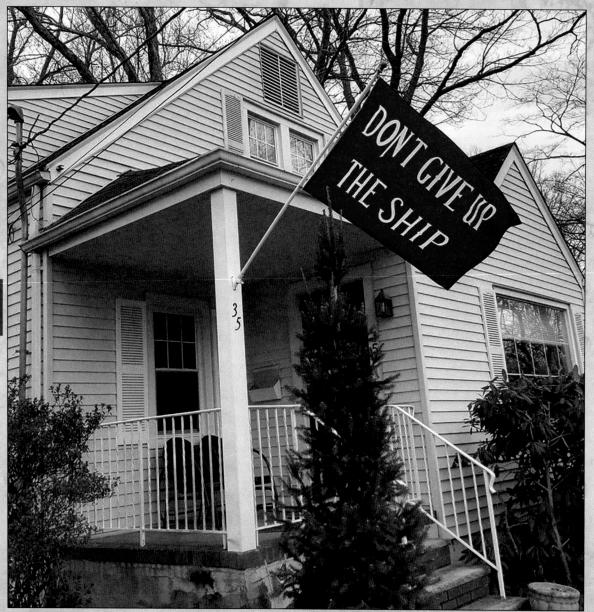

Flying High
A flag on a home in suburban Allendale, New Jersey lifts the
spirits of passersby, May 2020 (Photo by Lorraine Ash)

My Wake-Up Call

Terri deLyon

Early March 2020

've been a proud EMT for twenty-five years. When I began riding, the most serious threats to healthcare providers in the field were HIV and hepatitis. We rarely received word that a patient we transported was positive for either dangerous disease. Still, we had annual training on bloodborne pathogens and, for our protection, we took precautions with every patient.

For years warnings of new threats came and went without making much impact in our tiny suburb. We trained for outbreaks of West Nile virus, SARS, bird flu, H1N1, Ebola, Zika, and measles. We saw a few cases or suspected cases of each. Mostly, though, we settled into a comfortable routine of learning, readiness, and anticlimactic resolution.

When news broke in early 2020 that a new ailment was spreading rapidly throughout China and inching into Europe, I attended an infectious diseases review at our local hospital. At that point there were no confirmed cases in the US. Nevertheless, my EMS colleagues were wary. It's hard to scare emergency personnel; we're trained and practiced at controlling our emotions in times of stress and confusion. Yet I could tell by the types and tone of the questions being asked in the meeting that I wasn't the only one who felt uneasy.

Weeks passed. Warnings went out about patients presenting with flu-like symptoms who'd recently traveled abroad. Everyone glued themselves to news reports and listened to expert opinions on television. The captain of our Closter Volunteer Ambulance and Rescue Corps sent frequent emails to keep us informed, but the coronavirus still wasn't "real" to me.

My wake-up call arrived one night during my regular weekly duty shift. We were dispatched to a local address for someone feeling ill—a routine call I'd answered countless times. When I parked the rig at the curb, a police officer barked through his mask that the patient had recently returned from a trip overseas and was complaining of stomach pain.

I looked up and saw the patient being escorted to the ambulance. My heart dropped. He was pale. Between moans of pain, he gasped for air. His T-shirt was saturated with sweat, and he could not walk without assistance. My crewmate and I stared at one another for a beat before we both reached for the N95 masks under the counter and sprang into action.

Behind my mask, I felt disbelief, shock, self-doubt, and even panic, setting in. The man was not the sickest patient we'd ever treated. Not even close. What terrified me was what he represented.

After we delivered him to the emergency room for COVID testing and further evaluation, my mind raced. We wouldn't know for a few days whether he tested positive. I resolved to keep my distance when I returned home to my loved ones. For the first time in my EMS experience, I questioned, *Why am I risking exposing myself and my family to this disease? Why am I volunteering to do this?*

I looked back at all the times we'd drilled for a worst-case scenario that never came. They were history. The protective bubble had burst, blurring the lines between the hypothetical and the real. It could have happened anytime, but that day it happened to me and my crew. COVID was seemingly in our town, and we were among the first to stare it in the face.

As it turned out, another municipality a few miles to our south, Teaneck, became the epicenter of the disease in Bergen County. Other communities had many more confirmed cases than Closter.

Over the next three months I kept volunteering, responding to calls around my work-from-home schedule. I encountered COVID-positive and COVID-suspected patients, along with a steady stream of other emergencies. I can't say the fear of exposing myself or my loved ones has completely gone away, but it isn't as palpable as it was that first night.

The world has changed for essential workers. A lot has been said about how the COVID crisis affects our mental health even now. At times like these never forget that behind the mask of every essential medical professional is a person, just like you.

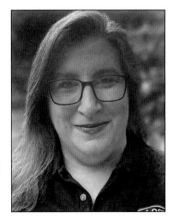

Terri deLyon is a wife, mother, full-time public school teacher, and emergency medical technician for Closter Volunteer Ambulance and Rescue Corps in Bergen County, New Jersey.

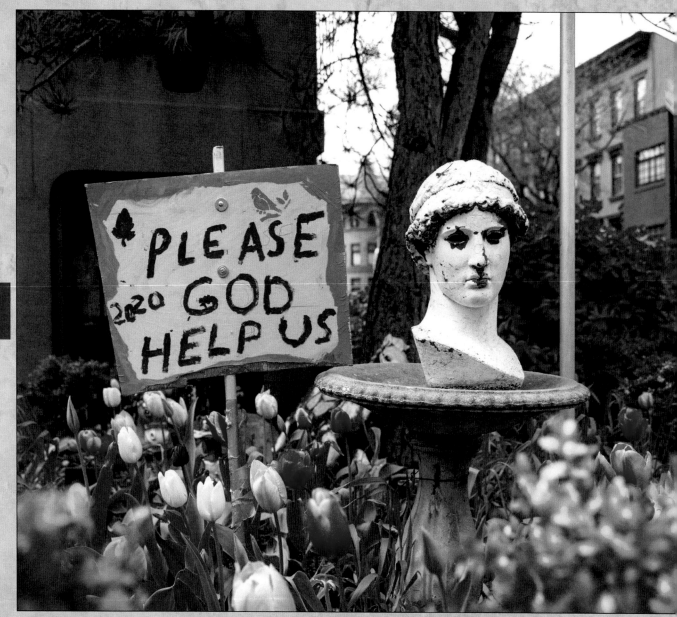

Urban Prayer
Brooklyn, April 16, 2020 (Photo by Walter Wlodarczyk)

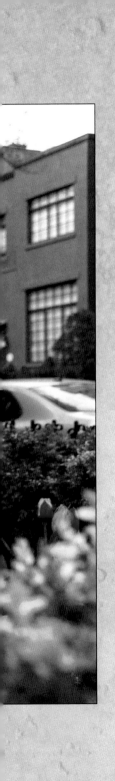

The Days the World Changed

Karen L. Phelps

Friday, March 20, 2020

Before I got out of bed this morning, I prayed for the nurses, doctors, and healthcare workers. I do that every morning. The number of people with coronavirus in Westchester County climbs higher and higher. I record the daily numbers on my kitchen calendar.

On Tuesday Governor Cuomo announced 25 percent of workers should stay home. On Wednesday it was 50 percent. Today everyone stays home except essential workers. All nonessential stores are closed—drastic measures to halt this deadly virus. Sports venues, movie theaters, libraries, and Broadway, all closed. Unthinkable.

I'm grateful for the girl who rings up my groceries. Who would have thought grocery store cashiers were essential? I thank her for working. She is surprised.

The line to get into BJ's is impossible. People are hoarding paper towels and toilet paper. How much toilet paper can you use?

At rush hour the roads are empty. It's eerie.

Saturday, March 21, 2020

It is spring now and the world as we know it has changed. *Everyone* is affected. For me, there are no more early morning writing sessions over breakfast at **Panera**. I practice social distancing, a new phrase, which means keeping six feet apart from everyone.

Many small businesses are forced to lay off workers. New York State unemployment is sky-high and the website to apply for benefits is so overloaded, it crashed. The number of people using food banks doubled, then tripled. What a nightmare for those scrambling to provide groceries. I am grateful to be retired with a fixed income so I can buy food.

For fear of spreading the virus, people are forbidden to gather now, which impacts my little church in Yorktown. Beginning Sunday, our pastor will give his sermon live on Facebook. They will remain posted for anyone who misses them.

Wednesday, March 25, 2020

I went to the vet with Keri, my collie, to ensure her broken leg is healing well now that the cast is off. I called the office from the parking lot. A girl came out with a plastic bag containing rubber gloves and a disposable paper mask. I had trouble getting the mask on. I was all thumbs. Inside everyone but the vet was wearing a mask.

The office was shorthanded so I was there two-and-a-half hours.

Tuesday, March 31, 2020

No international flights. People trying to get back home to the US are stranded all over the world.

Thursday, April 9, 2020

My sister, Mayona, sent me two handmade cotton masks—one a tie, the other with elastic. Elastic is impossible to get now because so many people are making masks. Mayona has made more than one hundred fifty masks for her large posse of friends. One woman requested that Mayona not make her mask from orange or yellow fabric because she doesn't look good in those colors. Talk about screwed-up priorities!

My friend, Jeanne, didn't have a mask. I asked my sister to send her one. She did. Jeanne later mailed her money.

Am I living through a sci-fi novel or *Twilight Zone* episode?

Thursday, April 16, 2020

I watched Governor Cuomo's daily briefing on TV, as I do every day. He is the voice of leadership and reason in this chaos.

Today I drove to the Croton ShopRite at 8:30 a.m. There was already a line around the block. Everyone stood six feet apart. I couldn't see the end of the line. Scary. I left because I can't stand in line for a long time. After all my surgeries, I'm too tired and can't breathe. Heart pounding, hands shaking, I drove back to the Yorktown Acme. No line! I was in and out fast. Thank God!

Alcohol sales are up 50 percent and domestic violence is rising.

Starting tomorrow, everyone in New York State is required to wear a mask if they are closer than six feet from another person. In other words, if you go into a store, you must wear a mask.

Thursday, May 14, 2020

Shocking news. On May 4 Stacie died from COVID-19. She and I participated in the same Friday writing critique group for several years. As a playwright, she often brought copies of short plays for us to read out loud. Any time Stacie commented on my writing, I took notes. Her comments were always on point.

Stacie, who left behind a husband and teenage twins, is the first person I know who died from COVID-19. Today I cried. For me, the virus now has a face and a name.

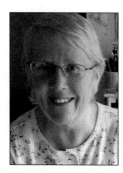

Karen L. Phelps is the author of *Maryann's Appaloosa,* a young adult novel, and *I Loved Them First,* a memoir in poetry and photos about the horse and collies who shared her life. The memoir was a finalist in the 2013 Dog Writers Association of America contest, her third DWAA award. She lives in Westchester County, New York.

Suddenly Sick

Laura Carriere

When the first announcements of a strange new virus called COVID-19 hit New York City's news, I was working. We allergy/immunology nurses stopped what we were doing and watched the Channel 7 broadcast with fear. At that point in January, the first case was being reported in the United States. I explained to the other nurses that I'd been working in infectious diseases when Ebola hit the US.

"This feels similar," I said, noting that Ebola was quickly contained. "We had more deaths from the influenza that year than Ebola itself."

We resumed working, hoping this situation would be similar.

March 15

I wake up with gastric symptoms and a fever. I'd drunk a bit the night before and had Blue Ribbon fried chicken a bit too late, an unusual combination for me. Another nurse I work with, who had shared the meal and drinks with me, wakes up with similar symptoms. As of now, the CDC is only reporting three symptoms for COVID-19—cough, fever, and shortness of breath. I'm already asthmatic and know I have no respiratory symptoms, but I still stay home from work for a week. The symptoms continue.

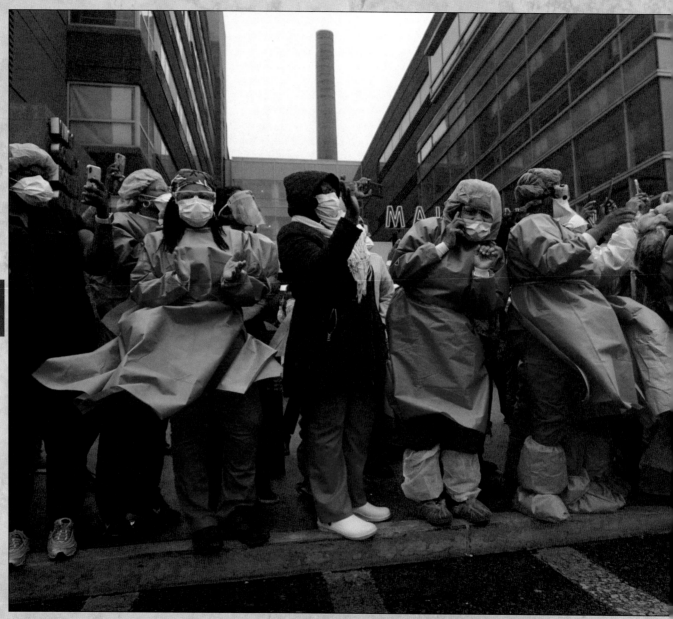

Appreciation
Nurses wave and clap outside Kings County Hospital in East Flatbush, Brooklyn as the New York Police Department honks and cheers for them during a drive-by salute, April 13, 2020 (Photo by Lloyd Mitchell)

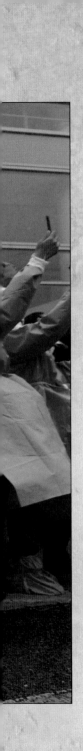

March 22

I wake up coughing, wheezing, and short of breath. My fever has spiked again after being absent for a couple of days, so I head to an urgent care center. I explain to the physician there that I was informed the day prior that a nurse and a physician I work closely with tested positive for COVID-19 in the past week and that another physician is awaiting results. He states he feels I have the coronavirus but will not swab me due to lack of testing. Besides, he says, the treatment would be the same anyway—fluids, rest, Tylenol.

March 25

I wake up feeling like my lungs are working extra hard. My fever has reached 103.7. I contact my director of nursing and the allergist/immunologist I work directly with. Both advise me to head to an ER. I arrive at a hospital in downtown Manhattan just as the Motrin I took is breaking my fever. I know this because I'm profusely sweating. My Albuterol has taken effect as well, as my breathing does not feel as labored. I look around and see patients in worse distress than I'm in, so I know I will not be admitted. I am put on the antibiotic Azithromycin, given IV fluids, and sent home.

March 27

I am coughing up bright red blood. My chest is heaving with every breath. Neither of my two inhalers is helping and my fever has spiked to 104.5. Both my superiors are now begging me to call 911, as it is clear I need to be hospitalized. I am hesitant because I have never stayed overnight in a hospital before, but I can feel my body shutting down systemically, so I dial 911 and am rushed by ambulance to a hospital in Brooklyn.

March 28

At 5 a.m. a physician comes to tell me my nasal swab is positive for COVID-19, as I already knew. He then throws me off-guard by asking if I have family in the nearby area. I should call them, he says, and tell them I love them, tell them what's going on with me. I am so scared, I text my fellow nurses, not my parents, because I want a second opinion and know a shift change is happening in a mere two hours. I am on 15 liters of oxygen and still heaving. My fever remains high and they are not giving medication. They forget to give me an IV until I remind them at 6 a.m. I have now been there for nine hours. At 8 a.m. I'm told I will be moved to the ICU. At 3 p.m., still in an overcrowded Critical Care ER, they tell me there is no bed for me and they need to find another ICU in New York City somewhere. Every hospital they call is completely full. They finally locate an ICU bed in the Bronx, forty-five minutes away. I have to get transferred and the oxygen tank cannot give me the amount I've been receiving for the transfer. I am not warned. I only know this from my own medical knowledge.

March 29

At 12 a.m. I arrive at the Bronx hospital gasping for air, only to be told my ICU bed was given away. I am then put on a newly renovated geriatric psych unit that hasn't even had patients yet. I am put in a room with no oxygen attached to the wall, just a completely bare room. Not even a trash can. They are trying to find a large oxygen tank for me, as I keep running out. This is not an ICU unit and this is the first time I feel I may die. I don't sleep. My fever spikes again. I cough up red blood.

They are not feeding me by 9 a.m. and I last ate on Friday, March 27. I just want cold water. I ask for some. It comes two hours later. Someone in full PPE comes into my room and steals my oxygen tank. I am gasping for air for five to ten minutes. They bring it back. It happens again—for more than ten minutes. I am trying to yell that I can't breathe, but no one can hear me in an isolation room with no call button. I am choking. I know I will die tonight if I am not moved out off this floor immediately. At 7 p.m. I start to choke on blood. I feel my lungs shutting down as well as my kidneys, my whole body. I press and press the newly made call button. No one comes for over an hour. I know a normal adult's O2 saturation levels should be 98–100 percent. Mine are now at 86 percent while on oxygen, then drop to 80 percent.

They call the ICU. I'm rushed down and put in a glass isolation room with all of the ICU physicians and nurses crowded around me. The doctor says he needs to intubate me immediately. I say no. He states they will watch me for an hour and if I can keep my O2 levels above 90 percent, they will not intubate me. I spend an hour staring at the wall, practicing deep, slow breathing while clutching my necklace that stores my only sister's ashes. I make the decision then and there that my parents will not go to a hospital and pick up another dead child with tubes down her throat. I succeed in keeping my O2 sats above 90 percent, so the staff lets me rest.

March 30

I wake up to two medical researchers shoving a stack of papers in front of me. They ask me to sign my name to try an IV transfusion for a blinded clinical trial. They state no one will know if I receive a placebo, 200 milligrams or 400 milligrams of a medication called Kevzara, made by Regeneron. I recognize the pharmaceutical corporation, as they make a biologic medication I use daily at work. I've personally seen that medication dramatically change patient's lives. I accept. I receive. I am still considered critical at this point: high fever, diarrhea, dehydration, kidneys not functioning, and labored breathing while attached to an oxygen mask.

March 31

I feel a bit better. I am not coughing up blood anymore. My fever is lower.

April 1

I wake up with no fever. I am able to eat a little bit. I am able to talk a little bit.

April 2

I now know I will not die. No fever for two days. My nurses say I look so much better. Two physicians come in and ask why I refused intubation. I explained my family's last image of my thirty-year-old sister: she was dead on a hospital bed with tubes down her throat. When I arrived at the hospital back then, I had pleaded with the nurses to take them out of her and to clean the blood off of her so my parents didn't have to see her that way. They stated that since she overdosed at home and was so young, there would be an investigation and they could not touch her body. That image will be forever embedded in my brain. I told the doctors I would not allow my parents to go through it again. They stated that had been the smartest move because it saved my life. I was the sole survivor of the ICU on the night of March 29. The other five patients who were intubated before me died. They change their "intubate immediately" policy.

April 3

I can smell again. I am tasting certain foods. I speak with my voice to my parents for the first time. They cry. I don't tell them that I have no TV or window, that I just watch all day and night from my glass isolation room as bodies are rolled in, code, and rolled out with a sheet over them. I haven't cried yet.

April 4

Today I turn thirty-six. My ten girlfriends who I grew up with create a Dropbox video of them and their kids, across the country, singing me "Happy Birthday." I finally cry. A lot.

April 5

I am moved to a medical surgical unit, as they have dropped me down to 4 liters of oxygen and I am talking without my mask. Doctors and nurses come into my room to ask my story. I become some sort of phenomenon, mostly because this trial medication saved my life. Today is the first day my medical researcher will admit I did not receive the placebo and was given either 200 or 400 milligrams. She states my markers went up dramatically all week after the IV transfusion I received and the areas of my lungs with damage can be seen improving on my chest Xrays. My arms are bloodied and bruised from twice-a-day blood draws and I am sick of taking so many medications, especially the blood thinner injections to the stomach.

April 6

They take off my oxygen mask. An hour later they tell me I am having an early discharge. I am not prepared and know they should keep me another twenty-four hours, as per protocol with the oxygen. They state they are scared I will get another infection from the hospital and that I need to continue lying in bed all day while at home. No one sends me home with oxygen and I don't get a wheelchair. I have to walk for the first time in ten days. I'm so weak. The nurses cheer for me as I leave the unit. I cry uncontrollably.

On the street I see a nurse who took care of me in the ICU and cannot believe she recognized me with my mask on. We both cry and she states she thought I would never walk out of here alive, as most doctors and nurses have already told me. I take a forty-five-minute Uber ride back to my apartment. I have a bad asthmatic episode on my second-floor apartment stairs. I take my inhaler a couple of times. I run into the shower. My roommate helps me stand as I scrub all the tape and electrode pad residue off me.

It has taken me more than two months to recover. I am still not at work but hope to be by July. I had to do a lot of breathing exercises in the beginning and was sleeping fourteen to more than eighteen hours a day, due to chronic fatigue and not sleeping for more than three hours straight in the hospital. I am now able to take small walks around the block and not use my rescue inhaler. I continue to read articles about lengthy recoveries from other healthcare providers who also almost died and who, like me, were also immunocompromised prior to getting COVID-19. I have hope and faith I will return to work soon to help the sick people of New York City, the reason why I got into this profession.

Laura Carriere is a nurse working and living in Brooklyn, New York. She has been a nurse for fourteen years and is currently attending a CUNY college to further her education.

FRONT LINES

The virus revealed the weaknesses in our healthcare system and many heroes who stepped forward to meet needs—first responders who kept riding, knowing they risked death; doctors and nurses who cared for the sick and dying, sometimes at terrible cost; bicyclists who rode empty city streets to deliver medical supplies and groceries. And there were more: store clerks, gas station attendants, teachers. Heroes showed up everywhere.

VOICES FROM AN EPICENTER Page 29

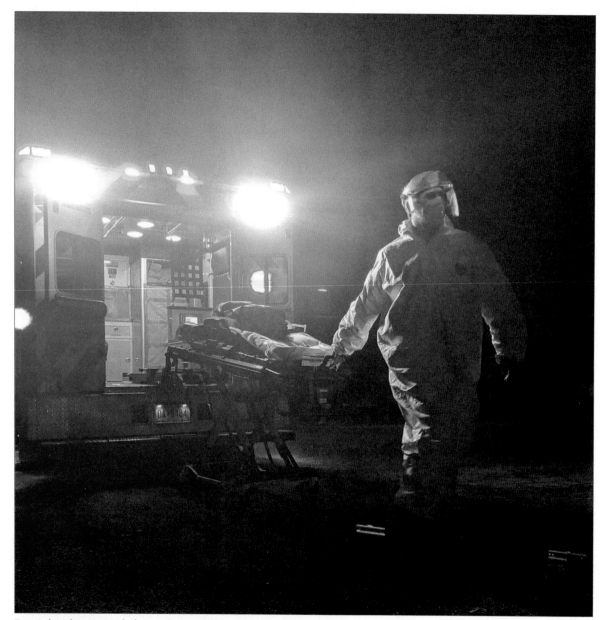

Teaneck Volunteer Ambulance Corps (TVAC) member Joe Horowitz
preparing the stretcher for a COVID-19 patient, April 11, 2020
(Courtesy of the Teaneck Volunteer Ambulance Corps)

Volunteering on the Very Front Line

Jacob Finkelstein

June 16, 2020

'll admit it. At first I was skeptical. I'd been hearing about the coronavirus outbreak in Wuhan but never seriously entertained the idea it would ravage my local suburban neighborhood in northern New Jersey. Boy, was I wrong.

Having joined the Teaneck Volunteer Ambulance Corps (TVAC) in 2012 at age seventeen, I'd been on a few thousand emergency calls and seen some crazy stuff. But never could I have imagined challenges we faced during the peak of the COVID-19 outbreak.

On Wednesday, March 11, we had our first COVID-19 patient. On Thursday we had our second. By Friday we had treated and transported ten COVID-19 patients. At the same time about half our normally active members stopped riding due to the virus—some because of their own health conditions, others because of a loved one's condition. I moved out of my house to avoid infecting my family.

From mid-March through April, our numbers skyrocketed. While we normally handle between twelve and fifteen calls a day, we were handling between twenty-five and thirty. Half the volunteers were covering double the number of calls.

And each call was physically and mentally exhausting—the time needed to gown up in full Personal Protective Equipment (PPE), the difficulty breathing in an N95 mask while carrying someone down a flight of stairs, the struggle to see while our face shields fogged up, the extra time and effort needed to properly disinfect every single ambulance surface, the continuous call after call after call, and the long waits at crowded hospitals.

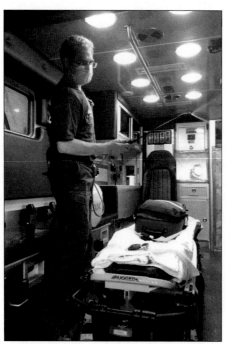

TVAC member Adi Segal disinfecting the patient compartment of an ambulance, May 4, 2020 (Courtesy of the Teaneck Volunteer Ambulance Corps)

Everything had changed at the hospitals. Giant tents filled with stretchers filled the spots where ambulances normally parked. People stood outside, hoping to get tested for COVID. Inside the ER lines of ambulance crews waited to get bed assignments for their patients. At first we were sent to a section of the ER sealed off with temporary walls and plastic sheets. Quickly, though, it got to the point where COVID patients filled the entire ER. Some patients with difficulty breathing or low O2 saturations were sent to the waiting room for up to ten hours.

The system was overwhelmed. Nurses, doctors, techs, paramedics, and EMTs all looked the same and not only because of our matching outfits—scrubs, N95 masks, face shields, and caps. We all had the same look of fear and mental exhaustion in our eyes. Every time someone took a breath to suck in oxygen through their N95, their breath fogged up their face shields. Yet they badly needed that oxygen to keep up with the constant stream of severely ill patients, to keep from giving up in the everlasting nightmare of COVID-19. Those patients needed oxygen, too, but they couldn't get it because of the virus.

Yet our volunteers who were still riding stepped up to the plate and kept pushing through challenge after challenge. Even members unable to take calls helped in other ways: they obtained PPE, filed for grants, raised funds, and handled press relations. As chief, I could not have been prouder of them and their amazing response to the pandemic.

As the days passed, there was a major shift in the types of calls we got. Initially we had patients experiencing "flu-like" symptoms. They had minor symptoms and were better off staying at home. While many of them healed on their own, we then started seeing patients we'd already treated. While they'd had a cough or fever the first time, they were experiencing severe respiratory distress the second time. Often their condition was grave. We had patients pronounced dead at the scene of the call in record numbers. As an organization,

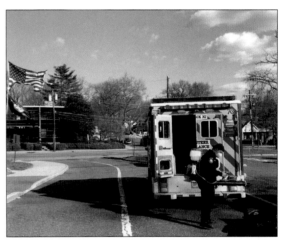

Jacob Finkelstein using hospital grade disinfectant in a modified leaf blower to clean an ambulance, April 1, 2020 (Courtesy of the Teaneck Volunteer Corps)

we normally see a handful of deaths in a month. During COVID-19 I saw five in one day!

Many of our members became infected with the virus and were forced to stop riding. Some were hospitalized for extended periods. It pained me that there was so little I could do for them. Under any other circumstance I would have ensured these members were not alone in the hospital but strict no-visitor policies made that impossible. One member was released from the hospital after a stay of several weeks only to have his spouse hospitalized for COVID-19 and placed on a ventilator.

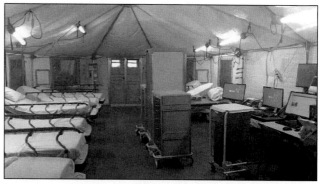

One of several tents prepared for the overflow from the Emergency Department at Hackensack University Medical Center, March 31, 2020 (Courtesy of the Teaneck Volunteer Ambulance Corps)

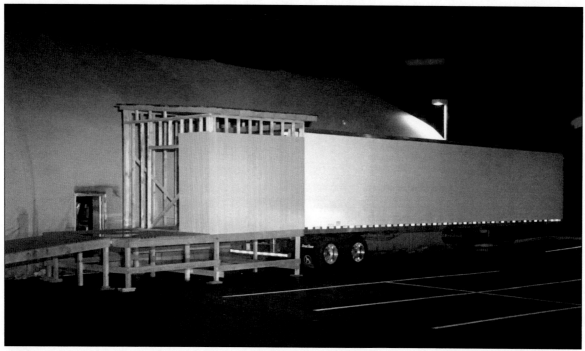

A refrigerator trailer parked at the Bergen County Emergency Complex being used to hold deceased bodies, April 13, 2020 (Courtesy of the Teaneck Volunteer Ambulance Corps)

Being a 100 percent volunteer organization, TVAC does not bill for any of our calls. We rely on donations from the greater Teaneck community. Our members not only volunteer their time but also incur expenses in order to serve on the corps. They purchase their own uniforms, EMT textbook, and medical equipment for their personal cars. In some cases they cover their own hospital bills. (Our members don't get the health insurance or benefits EMTs do in some towns.) They choose to make these sacrifices so they can save lives.

While recent months have been extremely challenging, we look forward to brighter days ahead. To partner with us in saving lives, visit teaneckambulance. org/donate.

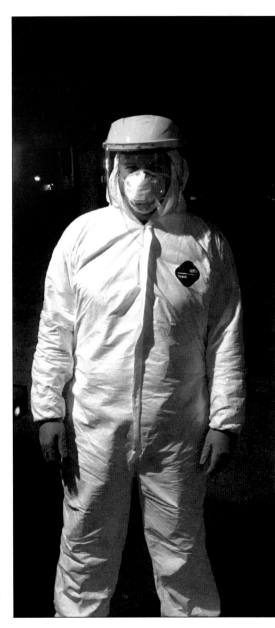

Jacob Finkelstein in full PPE after treating a COVID-19 patient, March 31, 2020 (Courtesy of the Teaneck Volunteer Ambulance Corps)

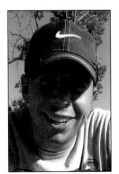

Jacob Finkelstein is chief of the Teaneck Volunteer Ambulance Corps, an all-volunteer organization that responds to more than forty-five hundred emergency calls a year.

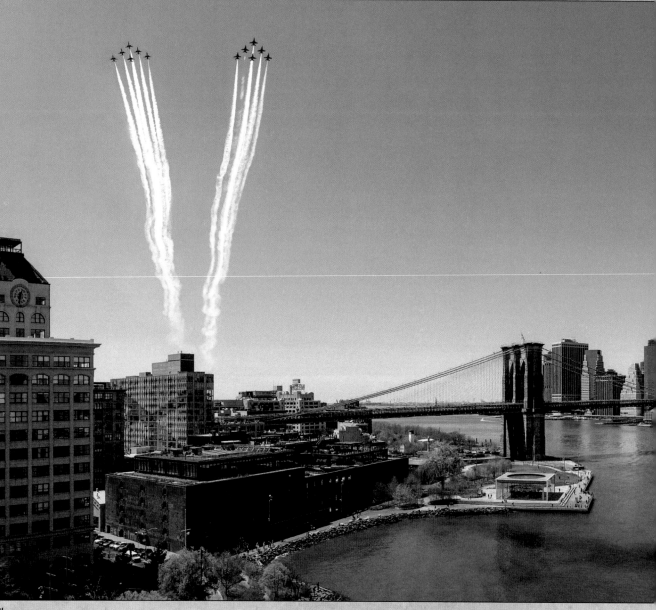

CORONA
CITY
Page 36

Flyover
The Navy's Blue Angels and the Air Force's Thunderbirds fly in formation over New York City
to honor all frontline workers against COVID-19, April 28, 2020 (Photo by Matthijs Noome)

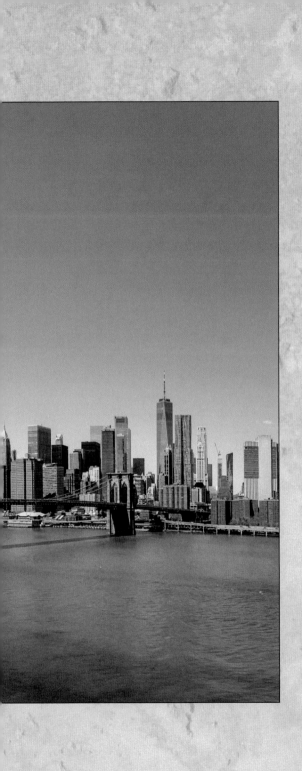

Battle Scars

Ruzha Skoblar

June 6, 2020

Somewhere in the distance I hear news of an illness spreading in China. *This must be like Zika or Ebola,* I think. *It's far away and doesn't threaten us in the US.* As an education specialist, I'd spent hours a couple of years earlier training staff teams on how to properly don and doff for these illnesses. Thankfully, there were few cases. I assumed COVID-19 would behave in the same short-lived way.

How quickly things changed mid-March. First, we had one patient who tested positive for COVID-19. To ensure the safety of the staff on that unit, I trained them in the proper use of personal protective equipment (PPE). Then another patient tested positive. And another. Then twenty, fifty, then hundreds.

My department taught class after class filled with scared nurses, ER doctors, respiratory therapists, and environmental staff. Over and over, they asked, "What should we do to care for these patients and protect ourselves?"

As the number of COVID-19 patients grew, we dedicated more units to their care. One day units designated for orthopedic patients were converted to COVID-19 units. The next day we converted surgical stepdown and oncology units. The changes continued daily until patients with this unseen, silent, deadly disease occupied most units. Even our cafeteria was converted into a seventy-four-bed COVID unit.

As the days progressed and patients' conditions worsened, the need for critical care beds exploded. I rounded on these units, previously designated for general medicine or surgery. They were filled with multiple pumps, code carts, and red bins, all indicating the presence of very sick patients. It was a sight I'll never forget.

Though amazed at how quickly the disease encased our whole hospital, I was even more amazed by the staff's resilience. We had trained them on one way of using the PPE. The situation became more critical, though, and PPE was in shorter supply so, following Centers for Disease Control and Prevention (CDC) guidelines, we taught them to clean and reuse some of it. During the height of the pandemic we developed nine methods to ensure proper procedures were followed. They applied to all areas of care.

Nurses became experts at bundling care, using MRI tubing as extension so they could more safely care for their patents without putting themselves at risk, and using various devices. To prevent central line infections, for instance, we used stat locks and large metal clips to keep IV tubing off the floor. To visualize patients in rooms without windows on doors, we used baby monitors.

We also became experts in proning (placing patients on their belly) and created "prone teams." There was no complaining, only a feeling of "go with the flow." I was so proud to be a nurse.

The strength of the human spirit was evident as nurses at bedsides struggled daily to care for patients and their families physically, emotionally, and spiritually. I was particularly touched by the plea of one ICU nurse as she sat outside the room of her ventilator-dependent patient. The patient's son had frantically called all day to ask about his mother's condition. Understanding their time was short, the nurse used the mother's limp finger to help her access her cell phone and dial her son's number. The conversation was brief but life changing. The mother's reaction told the nurse everything. No amount of sedation or illness could overcome the joy on her face at the sound of her son's voice. I felt chills as she spoke. The same nurse had an additional plea.

"Many patients come to the hospital with their cell phones," she said, "but they don't bring their chargers, leaving them without the ability to stay in touch with their family, adding to the stress and frustration."

I couldn't get her plea out of my head. I emailed my family and close friends and requested that they purchase the most common chargers. Their response was overwhelming. I was able to deliver almost two hundred chargers to these patients.

We're now at the pandemic's tail end with fewer than a hundred diagnosed patients. Many nurses, including my colleagues, have been sick. Some have lost loved ones. Yet they returned to work fiercely determined to do whatever it took to provide the best care.

I've been fortunate not to have lived through a war, but I am sure history will record the COVID-19 pandemic as one. We will carry scars from this battlefield. That is certain. What I will always remember, though, is that human resilience rises above all adversity. And it creates new hope we can use to prepare for the next war.

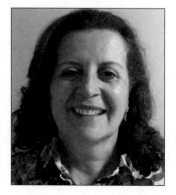

Ruzha Skoblar, MPH, BSN RN-BC, has been a registered nurse for thirty-five years. For more than twenty, she has worked as an education specialist at Hackensack Meridian Health. Her passion is teaching nurses and helping them understand that the care they provide to their patients every day can change the world.

A Good End

Geralyn Ponzio

As the pandemic began, I returned to our local hospital and offered my services. I'd worked there for ten years as a hospitalist and then moved on to outpatient medicine. I still did occasional shifts there, as needed, though. I am a physician with experience in internal medicine as well as palliative care.

I'd been hoping for a few extra shifts per week. The job I found that day exceeded my expectations. The need for a palliative care physician was urgent. COVID patients were pouring in the doors, and many were not going to make it. The hospital needed a physician to help its palliative care nursing team, which was fielding an onslaught of family questions about survivability, options, expectations, and death.

"We need you to start rounding with the ICU team and take over family discussions for the complex cases," I was told.

I took the position.

Two cases landed on my plate immediately. I reviewed them carefully. My colleagues told me how communications had broken down with these families. In one case, the family of a vibrant younger woman near death could not accept her loss. In the other, the family of an elderly woman, declining despite days of critical care, felt threatened when the hospital pushed for end-of-life discussions. Via phone and FaceTime, I needed to help both families understand the same impending outcome.

So began nearly three months of an experience I never expected. I showed up first thing every day of the week as the consults flowed in. My workdays quickly expanded to ten hours as I handled multiple complex cases. Often I returned to the hospital multiple times per day. I did whatever was required to offer hope while helping families realize "hope" sometimes meant a good death with a loved one present. My goal was not to convince every family to let go. It was to help them understand the situation and choose appropriately from an entire spectrum of choices.

Many a situation quickly changed. One day a family was told, "We will do everything in our power to keep her alive." The next day they might hear, "She is dying despite our best efforts. She will pass whether you want this or not, whether you are here or not. Please come be with her and let us do everything possible to make her comfortable. You will remember this your entire life. It will mean the world to both of you."

Our ICU is on the ground floor. Families denied entrance gathered in the gardens outside their loved ones' windows—a beautiful and unsettling practice we'd never seen before. Their faces pressed up against the glass, they watched helplessly. Our amazing nurses posted the patients' names in the windows so families could find the right room. Family members cried, wrote us messages on paper, and followed our every move through those windows as we hustled in and out, caring for patients.

For some families whose loved one survived, I played a more supportive background role. Survivors often were left with several complications and complexities.

I navigated conference and video calls daily and text conversations all day and night. I spoke with state guardians and interpreted Spanish for the families of ICU patients from other countries as they signed for treatments and listened to medical staff. Sometimes I just rolled up my sleeves and helped the ICU physician do their job when they needed it. I ordered treatments and placed central lines.

As I helped support both life and death, I sometimes found myself at odds with other physicians' concepts about death and dying. At times families disagreed with our recommendations entirely and pushed full steam ahead for recovery, often at a heavy cost. Some of their loved ones spent their last days alone and struggling to breathe, despite the ventilator.

I'm proud of the work we did and of my colleagues, including nurses, respiratory therapists, and housekeepers. For everyone involved the challenge was enormous. It was a terrible time. But even after twenty years in medicine, I learned so much about life, death, and dying in such a short time.

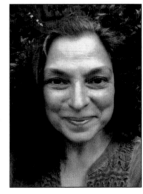

Geralyn Ponzio, MD, is a board-certified Internist with a subspecialty in hospice and palliative care medicine. She now works in primary care in eastern Pennsylvania and northern New Jersey. She continues to moonlight at her local hospital as needed and hopes to expand palliative care services there for her community.

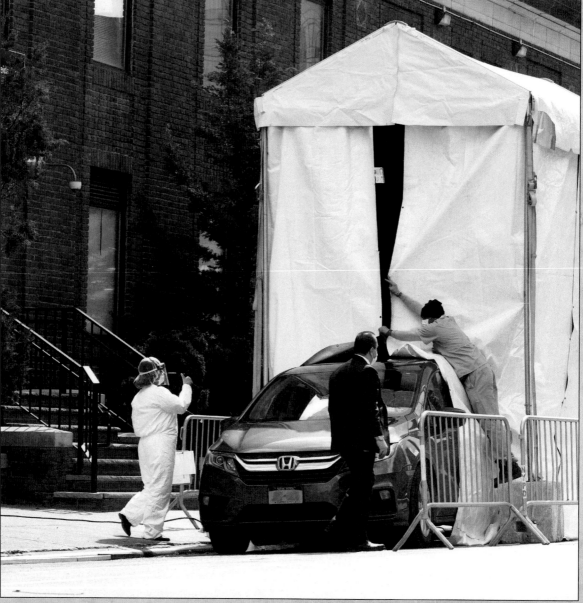

Ubiquity of Death
Workers at Woodhull Hospital in Bushwick, Brooklyn, remove bodies of deceased COVID-19 patients to refrigerated trucks in a makeshift morgue, April 3, 2020 (Photo by Lloyd Mitchell)

What It Was Like

Maureen F. Bowe

June 2020

Numerous times over the past three months, people who know I'm a nurse have asked, "What's it like?" I immediately know what they mean: What's it like being on the front line of the COVID pandemic? Normally, I tell them it's been fine. Some days I ramble on. Most often, I simply say, "It's been tough." If I say more, I'm afraid the floodgates will open about what this pandemic has really been like for nurses like me.

I remember April 17, 2020 all too clearly. That was the day my colleague, Gabby, a registered nurse, left the hospital after recovering from COVID-19. Finally, after eight weeks of this pandemic, I had something to look forward to. First, I heard the clapping. Then came the sound of the staff singing, "Rise Up." Finally, I saw Gabby herself. Lesley pushed her wheelchair.

Gabby was surrounded by her coworkers. I started to cry. She passed me. I looked into her eyes. I was grateful then, as now, that she never required a ventilator but she'd come so close! I'd been so frightened that day to think one of our own would need this lifesaving equipment.

I looked out the lobby window. There was Gabby's mother, standing by their maroon car. My heart beat faster. *What if that was me waiting for Kelly, my beloved daughter? Would I be able to stand there so patiently?* Gabby was finally out the door and by her mother's side. They embraced. Gabby slowly got into her car.

It was my turn then to sit down in the hospital lobby and say a prayer. Thankfully, Gabby was one of the lucky ones who survived COVID-19. Not all will be so fortunate. This pandemic has been terrifying.

And here's what it really was like to live through the many scenarios of this crisis.

> *It was unfathomable to see a nurse holding an iPad to the face of a dying patient so their family could witness their loved one's death.*
>
> *It was frightening to witness my friend, the infection control practitioner, working seven days a week and hope she had the stamina to continue.*
>
> *It was unnatural to wear a mask from the moment I stepped into the hospital to the moment I left.*
>
> *It was unnerving to see grandparents cry because they missed the birth of their first grandchild.*
>
> *It was inspiring to observe nurses caring for their patients, their families, and their fellow nurses, exhausted after working sixteen hours straight.*
>
> *It was heart-wrenching to deny a family's request to visit a critically ill patient.*
>
> *It was challenging to be responsible for scheduling the correct number of healthcare workers to safely take care of our patients, knowing there was less staff than needed and realizing my colleagues were at risk for contracting COVID.*

It was unimaginable to create a ventilator surge plan while wondering if I'd be the one responsible for making a life-and-death choice on who would use this emergency equipment.

It was uplifting to see my staff protect their colleagues who were pregnant or immunocompromised by reducing their risk of COVID exposure.

It was scary to be called in the middle of the night by a friend whose three-year-old child may need to be admitted because of respiratory problems.

It was rewarding to witness staff helping each other and safely donning personal protective equipment.

It was horrifying to develop a triage process for hospitalized beds, knowing some patients wouldn't get one.

It was terrifying, gratifying but, most of all, awe-inspiring. I have never been more proud to say, "I am a nurse."

At the height of the COVID pandemic, nurses were at bedsides, as we have always been, caring for our patients, holding their hand, granting final requests, listening to their regrets, providing comfort, and making sure no one died alone. We know it's our legacy of caring and compassion that will inspire the next generation of men and women to want to say, "I am a nurse."

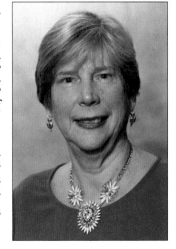

Maureen F. Bowe, MSN, RN, always wanted to follow in her mother's footsteps and become a nurse. Her dream was realized when she graduated from Thomas Jefferson University School of Nursing in 1974. She has never taken lightly her responsibility to care for others when they are the most vulnerable. She has always believed that being a nurse is an honor.

Brooklyn Bridge, April 11, 2020 (Photo by Walter Wlodarczyk)

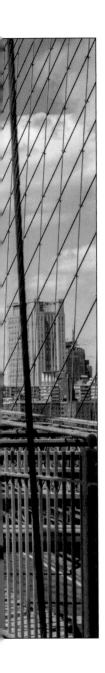

Pandemic Praxis

Dinah Gumns

May–June 2020

In mid-May my mother, a travel nurse, stopped by New York City on her way up to Rhode Island and stayed in midtown. It was her first time in the city. Homeless shelters were over-crowded. Hospitals weren't keeping patients overnight unless they had to. The summer heat had landed. All this, along with the lack of tourists, transformed midtown and Times Square back to its glory days of the late '70s.

We bid good morning back to a group of men smoking crack on Thirty-Sixth at 10 a.m., rounded Eighth, and grabbed some bagels and coffee. Then we split up for the day. I did my usual volunteer delivery runs on my bicycle for Corona Couriers, which provides free groceries to vulnerable populations; Last Mile PPE NYC, which provides N95 masks and face shields to health-care workers; and Make The Road NYC, which runs a food bank in Queens.

That evening my mother and I met up again around 10:30 p.m. and walked through an empty Times Square—two entire city blocks advertising products no one could buy to no passersby as homeless New Yorkers set up camp beneath the glow.

A few days later, the *New York Times* published the paper marking one hundred thousand deaths due to COVID while Southern states pushed for the right to reopen.

Two weeks later, the entire country erupted. Memorial Day openings caused massive outbreaks and yet another killing of an unarmed black man caused the largest global civil rights protest in history.

Meanwhile, the current administration continued to manipulate the virus into a political nightmare rather than address it as a basic public health crisis. And police brutality in the guise of enforcing social distancing, especially in New York, became undeniable. Seemingly hourly, videos circulated showing excessive force used on shoppers, people sitting on their stoops, or even bystanders in black neighborhoods. Reports came back that over 85 percent of those arrested for violating social distance orders were black and brown.

Within hours of Minneapolis protesting and demanding justice in their city, New York City responded in kind. No jobs, a bloated budget that doesn't serve the people of the city, and generations of injustice all converged and broke our sense of social decorum.

Both Corona Couriers and Last Mile asked those who participated in large protests to self-quarantine for two weeks afterward, before we continued delivering. Unfortunately, the Venn diagram of people who rally to provide basic services for free and people who show up *en masse* to demand their communities be safe from extrajudicial murder by the state is an overlapping circle.

Many of us are now delivering masks, water, and supplies to protesters instead. I'm now awaiting the results of my most recent COVID test before I start delivering for food banks again. Our shipment of masks is being diverted and supplied to harder hit areas now, so we're unable to fulfill orders for PPE despite the fact that New York City hospitals still need them badly.

The morning of June 25, I read that the country broke the record we set in April for new COVID-19 cases on any given day. As I rode my bicycle over the nearly empty Williamsburg Bridge, I glanced to the roadway beneath me. I peeked at the bumper-to-bumper rush hour traffic that spanned from the bridge entrance in Brooklyn to its exit in Manhattan. I rode past one of the streets where the morgue trucks used to dock, now full of maskless joggers.

Back at work now, I no longer volunteer full time to deliver essentials to medical workers and people in need.

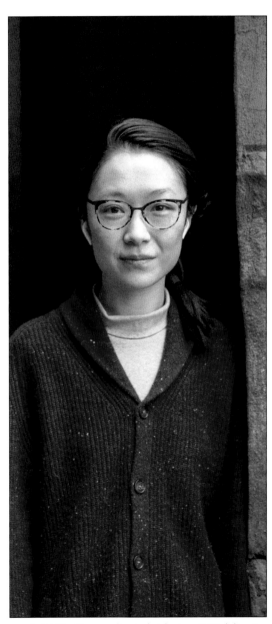

Artist Xin Liu coordinated volunteer PPE deliveries to essential medical workers at the peak of the outbreak in New York, April 2020
(Photo by Walter Wlodarczyk)

I can't wrap my mind around the events of the last five months. Each emergency gave birth to the next. Our collective denial and slow acceptance of that was bad enough. My fear lies in our quick dismissal and our desperate hope for a return to normal. I mean that for both the pandemic and the uprising around police brutality. The responses mirror each other: denial leading to begrudged acknowledgement, then acceptance and changed behavior by some and outright rejection by others. Next came the political polarization of something that is actually just about valuing human life and reducing harm—

wearing masks. We are pandered to with good public relations optics that belie absolutely no solutions. And now we yearn for permission to forget, or at least be exempt from the problems.

I am exhausted.

I used to tell myself that it was okay to run myself ragged, that doing so was temporary, that it won't always be like this. I reminded myself that the situation will ease, that the virus will die out, and we will make it out of this alive.

Now, I listen. I wait.

Our social state is not an inconvenience. It is a reckoning. We have seen the disparity between

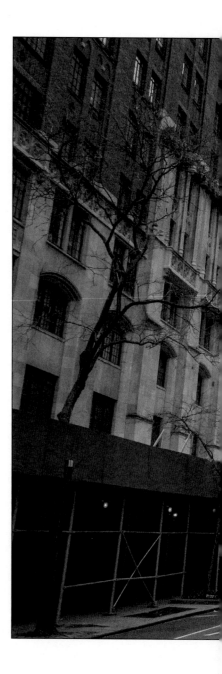

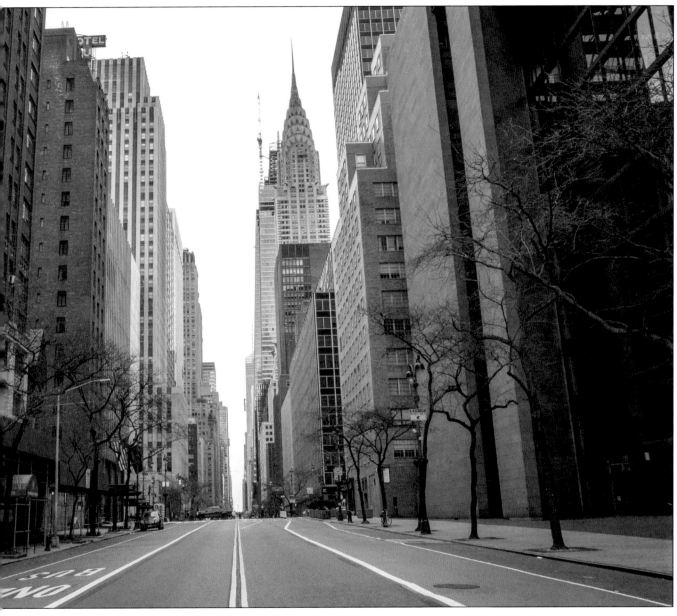

East Forty-Second Street, Manhattan, April 10, 2020 (Photo by Walter Wlodarczyk)

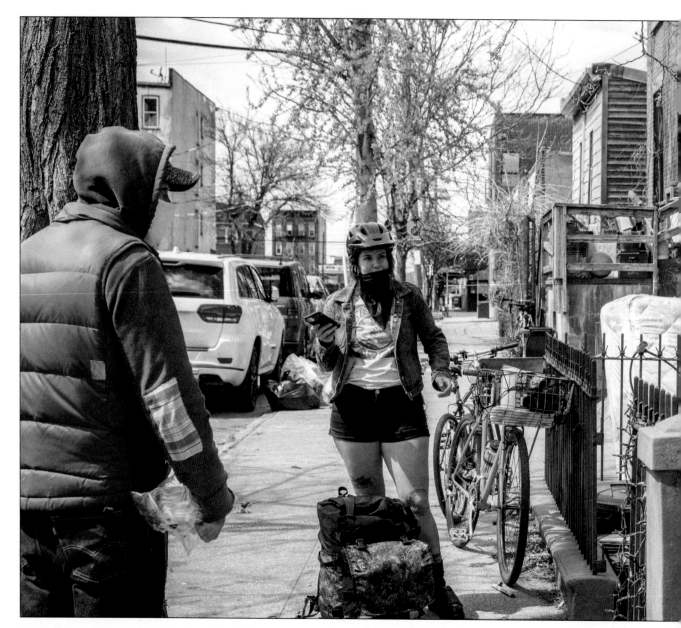

Dinah delivering PPE in Brooklyn, April 16, 2020
(Photo by Walter Wlodarczyk)

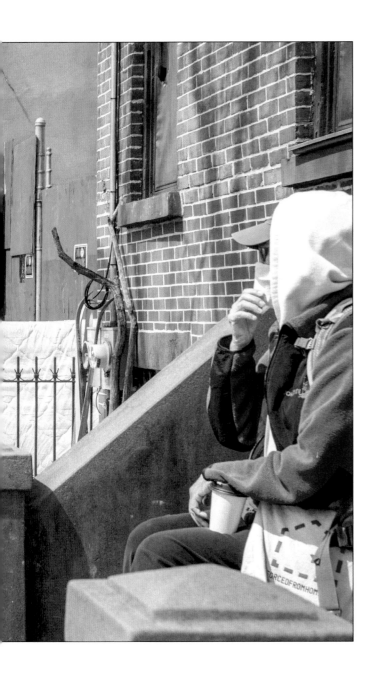

the world we want and the world we have. We know we are capable of living in a world where we are taken care of; we drew the blueprints back in March. And I am glad to be of service in whatever capacity I can.

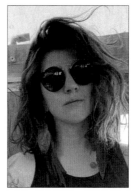

Dinah Gumns is a fabricator of things, tangible and not, in Brooklyn, New York.

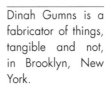

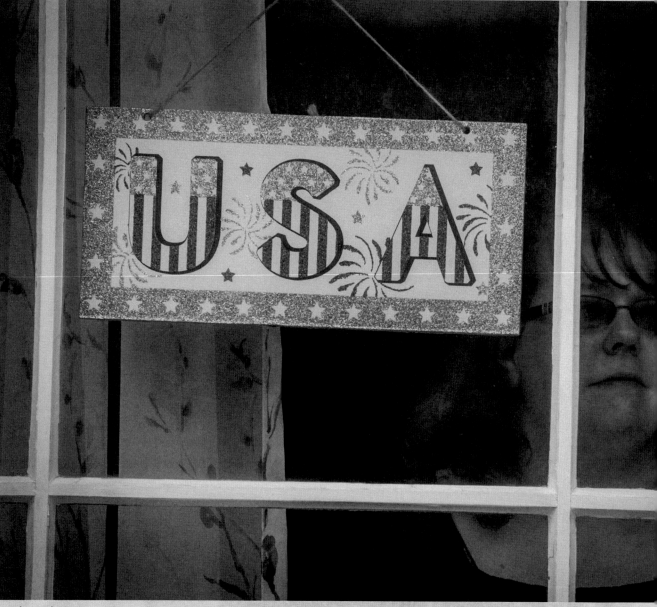

Inside Looking Out
A woman looks out the window of a nearby title business as about 100 residents gather at the
Monroe County Courthouse Square in Pennsylvania for an Open Now Rally Friday, May 15, 2020
(Photo by Daniel Freel)

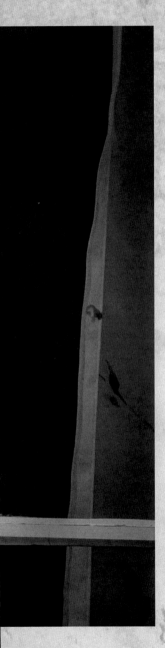

LOSSES

The mounting death toll overwhelmed and frightened us. Yet we also experienced each loss one person at a time, forgoing funerals for safety's sake and grieving alone. Every victim was more than a number on a chart to us. We were losing people we loved, the guardians of our history, talented medical workers, leaders, writers, artists, and musicians. We knew it would take years to fully understand such suffering and death.

VOICES
FROM AN
EPICENTER
Page 57

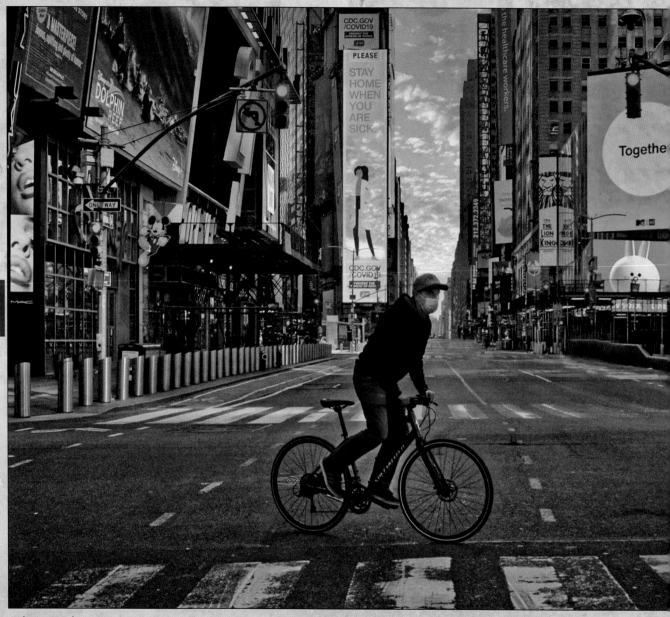

Solitary Cyclist
A lone cyclist bikes through an empty Times Square during the height of the COVID-19 quarantine, May 13, 2020
(Photo by Ellen Bedrosian)

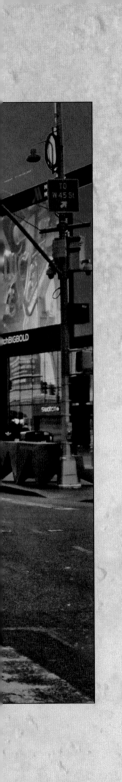

Another Twenty-Four Hours

Jolinda Hockaday

'␣ve lived alone for many years. But sheltering in place? A lockdown? What gives here? On March 15, 2020, our elected officials closed down the state, city, and town where I live. Since when does New York City close the MTA Long Island Rail Road for cleaning, disinfecting, or sanitizing? Since when do New York City schools shut down? Unheard of. Not even a hurricane shuts down the city that never sleeps. Even 9/11 shut the schools and airspace for just one day.

But COVID-19 was different. People were leaving the Earth in record numbers.

In March, April, and May, the same scene replayed itself over and over. The virus couldn't be contained. Childhood friends—some older, some younger, some the same age—were gone in an instant. One day I heard the news that one loved one had succumbed to the virus. A day later, there was another. Then another and still another, all within days.

The shock didn't wear off. My aunt in Cape Cod, my oldest son's godmother, fellow teachers from my school, loved ones from church, Sunday school teachers, assistant ministers, and pastors—all gone! Even my ex-husband, who works in a hospital, got the virus though his life was spared. He recovered miraculously.

All the death was no wonder, though. The Centers for Disease Control and Prevention eventually released statistics showing that Latino and Black people were three times as likely to become infected, compared to their white neighbors. They were also more than twice as likely to die from the coronavirus. And that's not just in New York City but around the whole country.

And there I was alone, quarantined. A recent retiree from the classroom, I was no longer with the students I loved and cherished so much.

On shutdown day I browsed online, looking for some inspiration. I came across the Empowered Living Community and footage of a live sunrise at Jupiter Island, Florida. I later learned the CEO of Empowered Living taped this majestic event from his balcony for forty-five minutes every morning, rain or shine. Every day, I tuned in. Recently, on June 27, my birthday, we completed the hundredth day of sunrises. What a blessing! Those sunrises have captivated me, almost hypnotized me.

I knew, too, I didn't watch them alone. The circle of club members grew from a few hundred the first few days to 1.8 million on my birthday. This event is governed by the laws of nature: the fireball in the sky appears on the blue-gray skyline that demarks the horizon. Meanwhile, the rhythmic sounds of the ocean lull me as the waves ebb and flow. Palm tree branches sway and bend in the gentle, and sometimes not-so-gentle, breezes off the ocean. Sea turtle eggs hatch on the sand. Quickly, the hatchlings crawl into the ocean, escaping birds looking for a meal.

All of us watching witness the work of the greatest designer, the greatest painter, the greatest artist and rejoice in the divine handiwork. We feel the breath in our lungs and give thanks. Together, we testify to the ocean's vastness and our own faithfulness that we will get this new day right. We have been given another twenty-four hours of life when so many did not wake up, open their eyes, or put their feet on the floor, did not see a new sunrise.

Jolinda Hockaday is a retired schoolteacher, a Toastmaster Competent Communicator, a mentor, and a motivational speaker. She is a John Maxwell certified coach and has served as an assistant instructor for the Dale Carnegie Course. She lives on Long Island.

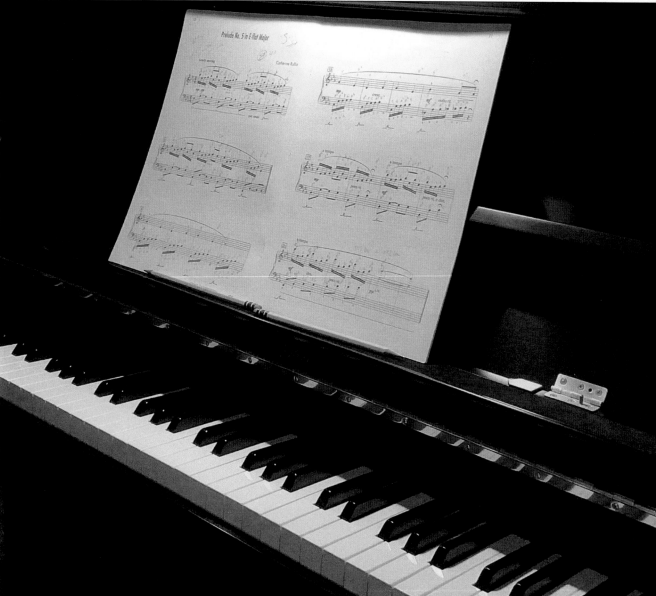

The Boston piano by Steinway & Sons, a saving grace and refuge, August 2020 (Courtesy of Linda Morales)

The Piano

Linda Morales

May 2020

That evening I sat at my piano. I had to prepare Burgmüller's "Arabesque" and Lady Allyson's "Minuet" for my master class and recital. The Virtual Piano Camp was going to start April 17. Already in lockdown for more than a month, I woke up almost every day afraid that if I breathed the wrong way, or if my chest felt too tight, I might be stricken by the invisible monster. And if I had it, might I, too, die?

Little did I realize that piano would become my refuge. Once I put my fingers on the keys, I entered another dimension.

I was supposed to have gone to the Summer Sonatina International Piano Camp in Vermont where thirty-two pianos awaited all of us. Immersed in a world of piano, all of us were to have spent a week away from the routines of daily life. We would have listened to one another during master classes, relished individual lessons with teachers, enjoyed piano talk and, at the end of the week, performed pieces from our repertoires for our recital.

But the world was suddenly different. We were all sheltered in place, working from home, socially distant.

I found myself playing "Prelude No. 5 in E-flat Major," a gentle moving piece by Rollin, over and over again. It helped me find solace amid the sad news I heard each day. The song also blocked the worrying sounds of ambulances on the Bronx streets. *Another soul being rushed to the hospital.* I said a prayer and continued to play. The gentle notes, played over the sounds of doom in the distance, soothed my fright.

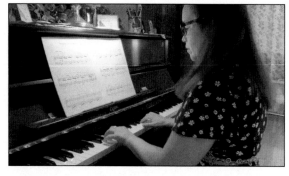

Linda Morales plays "Prelude No. 5 in E-flat Major," the piece that helps her find solace, August 2020 (Courtesy of Linda Morales)

Finally, virtual piano camp was launched and, after a few little Zoom glitches, everyone was online. Together, we escaped into the world of piano. But that just got me to thinking how I'd found piano camp in the first place.

I credit my boss for being my piano angel. When I celebrated thirty years at work, I was given time for a spiritual retreat. I was excited about the gift, especially since I went to a silent prayerful retreat each year. But when my boss found out I'd started taking piano lessons, he called me into his office.

"Why don't you go to a piano retreat instead of a silent retreat, for goodness' sake!" he said.

Next thing I knew, we'd found a piano camp in Vermont and I was on my way.

After virtual piano camp, I continued to practice. As the weeks cumulated and quarantined life became the new normal, I recorded a piece and sent it to my boss to enjoy. In spite of the virus, in spite of the world being upside down, in spite of having to work remotely, I found joy and comfort in playing. Every day, after Zooming for work, I came downstairs to practice. Many people continued to get word of loved ones being rushed to the hospital.

Then on Monday, May 18, I received a call. My boss was rushed to the hospital. He'd had trouble breathing. The next day he wrote to all of us on staff: "COVID didn't get me; just an infection. I'll be here through the weekend to clear it up."

I wrote him back, "We are Tough! We are Smart! Stay Vigilant!"

Immediately, I texted a dear friend who happened to be a doctor in the emergency room of the hospital. She selflessly went to see him on my behalf. She put on her protective gear, went back to the hospital, walked into his room, and found him sitting up, ready to eat.

She'd brought him a piece of cheesecake and a card from me. Besides introducing herself as one of the hospital's doctors, she explained she knew me from our rosary prayer group. He quickly interrupted her.

"Nice," he said, "but have you heard her play the piano?"

Three days later, on May 23, he took his last breath.

As I sit at the piano now, still shocked by the news, I play "Prelude No. 7 in B Minor" by Vandall. In his honor, I tell myself, *I must play on.*

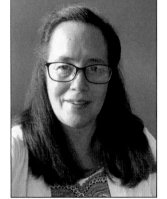

Linda Morales has worked for an international trade association for thirty-three years, organizing programs and conferences around the world. Outside work she has been very active in her church and house of prayer. Her hobbies include crocheting, writing, and piano. She resides in New York.

Sign Language
Homemade signs such as this one in Midland Park, New Jersey provide a community
feeling when everyone is isolated in lockdown, May 2020 (Photo by Lorraine Ash)

Lost and Found and Lost

Lorraine Ash

May 8, 2020

The long hand of COVID-19 snatched Barbara from our family. Barbara, one life of 8,952 lost, according to the latest death chart. Barbara, who I just found after untangling reams of genealogical records and crossing a desert of family estrangement. Barbara, who I was never supposed to meet.

In 2015 I called her husband, Gene, my cousin, and introduced myself. We decided to meet some weeks later at an Atlanta Bread on a highway. Barbara came to support him that day, standing by his side, pretty as a picture with short blonde hair and a red outfit. She extended her hand.

We all sat in a booth where she listened to us trade more than a century of stories and pictures. We filled in blanks for each other. I had a huge one. Barbara, mother of four, had met the grandmother I never knew. She understood the wound and scrambled for a connection.

"I have her roasting pan at home," she told me, her easy smile lighting up her face. "I use it every Thanksgiving. After all, she was Gene's aunt. Sometimes she came over to the house for picnics."

After decades of no contact, she produced the only tangible thing left to bridge three generations—a roasting pan. In the moment her acuity and sensitivity delighted me. Not everyone would have been as thoughtful or as willing.

"You must come to the house," she said. "We'll have lunch."

So a few weeks later I ventured to their house on a lake. At age fifty-six, for the first time, I set foot in a home from that side of the family. Just walking over the threshold felt magical and right. We sat in a room like an art gallery, eating a delicious gluten-free meal she'd lovingly prepared as Gene and I talked on. After a time, we moved past the ancestors and into our own lives—who we were, where we'd been, what we'd done. Just like a family does.

Even at eighty, Barbara, a painter, still worked in an art gallery. She loved her art. It was everywhere in their home. She loved her home. She loved her husband, her children, her grandchildren and, very clearly, her life. She had love to spare.

Just as she was to end a successful treatment program in a rehab facility, the virus came. Having no mercy for the weak, it killed her quickly. We'd had no past. It took our future. The news of her death jolted me. The jolt affirmed the connection, so I was glad to feel it.

Like a black wave, death had taken unreconciled family members for decades. No one was ever notified. No one cared to notify. Many times, news of a death would have been like news of the death of a stranger, anyway.

Like all the memorial services, Barbara's will be sometime in the future. Whenever it is, I will be there to mark her passing, to say goodbye, to say, "I knew her."

I started my quest to find my long-gone grandmother, who had abandoned her own children. Barbara had given me a piece of that long-lost past. But the truth is, she gave me more than my grandmother ever would have. She gave me a piece of herself. She stood in that terrible void and imbued it with her grace. And no virus can kill that kind of humanity.

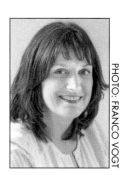

PHOTO: FRANCO VOGT

Lorraine Ash, MA, is a New Jersey-based book editor, author, and literary coach.

Ryan, Jessie, Madonna, and Nico enjoy time together on a cruise to the Caribbean, December 6, 2015 (Courtesy of Nico Ferreras, MD)

Family Physician, Family Man

Nico Ferreras, MD

My father, Jessie Ariel Ferreras, MD, worked a long weekend March 20-23, 2020. A family physician in Waldwick, New Jersey, he was very proud to be an everyday doctor who specialized in everything. The four-day stretch was no different as he tested many patients for COVID-19.

That Monday, upon his return from work, he didn't feel well. His own COVID-19 test had come back positive. Yet he sat at his home desk on March 24, and every day thereafter, with a long list of patients' names. Following each was a "+" or "-." One by one, he called to give them their results and instructions. That's the way he'd been with his patients for twenty-five years—devoted.

"If there's no improvement or if you have any concerns, don't hesitate to call the office," he always said.

On April 2, supposedly his tenth day with COVID symptoms, he had a fever but said he was fine, not short of breath. He had dinner and went to bed. So it was a shock when the next day, April 3, his health took a turn for the worst. He passed away at home in the arms of his loving wife and my mother, Madonna, a nurse. He was only sixty-two.

His passing marked the end of a short yet wonderful life. The eldest of six, my father grew up in Lumban, a small provincial town in Laguna, Philippines. From the start, he dreamt of becoming a doctor and serving those around him. Knowing the path wouldn't be easy, he worked tirelessly to make his dream a reality for himself and his family, friends, and future patients.

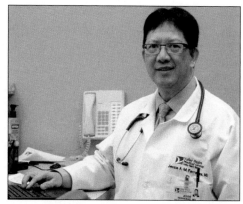
Typical day in the office for Dr. Ferreras
(Courtesy of Nico Ferreras, MD)

He studied medicine at the University of Santo Tomas Faculty of Medicine and Surgery (UST FMS). After graduating, he pursued medical training in the United States and completed his residency in family medicine at JFK Medical Center in Edison, New Jersey. He found a second home at work where he managed patients from children to the elderly and cases from the common cold to chest pain.

His clinical skills, ranging from suturing lacerations to ear irrigations and Pap smears, were matched only by his kindness and compassion. Everyone he came into contact with loved him. One of my father's colleagues called him a "trusted friend and the backbone of the office." Nurses admired his dedication. He often called patients on his free time, as he did the week before he died. He gave them lab results and updates; he knew they were waiting. He refilled prescriptions; he knew they needed their medications.

To patients, he was more than an approachable compassionate doctor who took his time to address their concerns. He was a friend, a shoulder to lean on, an extended member of the family.

And yet he was more than a family physician. He was a family man, happily married for thirty-two years. Even with a busy schedule, he found time to go to sporting events with me and my brother, Ryan, and to see Broadway shows with our mother. As a family, we traveled the world. He encouraged my brother and me to enjoy our lives and pursue careers we'd enjoy. Ryan, an avid hip-hop dancer, works as a software engineer. Like my father, I'm a doctor in family medicine.

I will never forget my beautiful upbringing, just as my father never forgot where he came from. In 2008 he and his siblings started a yearly family tradition: they donate a holiday meal to three hundred fifty families in Lumban so no one goes hungry during the Christmas season. He visited as often as he could and was very fond of family get-togethers and class reunions.

After his passing, my mother, brother, and I learned of hundreds of people who loved and cared about my dad. His medical school classmates created a Facebook tribute page and posted memories and pictures of him. On April 12, Easter Sunday, his coworkers and friends formed a drive-by procession in front of our house. They got out of their cars and, one by one, left pictures, flowers, cards, and candles in honor of Dr. Ferreras.

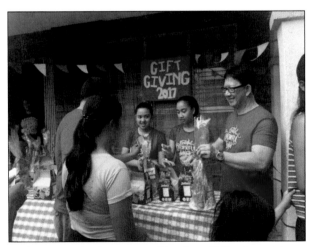

Dr. Ferreras in his hometown of Lumban, Philippines giving a holiday meal, December 2017
(Courtesy of Nico Ferreras, MD)

Beloved patients have sent cards and letters recounting memorable experiences. One wrote about her lack of follow-up from a specialist.

"Your father persisted," she said. "He did not give up calling me till he got a response. He told me I had pneumonia."

Another told the story of how Dr. Ferreras had helped in every aspect of his life for more than twenty years.

My dad's passing was made more memorable when people donated on his behalf. The money went to COVID-19 response efforts, including PPEs. He would have liked that.

Though COVID-19 took his life at the early age of sixty-two, he had checked off all the boxes for a meaningful life. He'd found his true calling, married his one true love, and seen his sons become men. He healed the sick, traveled the world, and made the lives around his better. He lives on through the lives he touched, so he goes down in history as a hero.

And I do my best to follow in his footsteps as the next "Dr. Ferreras," though, for now, hearing people address me that way always reminds me of him.

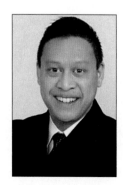

Nico Ferreras, 30, graduated Boston College and, like his father, earned his medical degree at UST FMS. He is currently a first-year resident in family medicine at Meadville Medical Center, Pennsylvania.

Memorial Day 2020

Jan Barry

Bury 'em six feet deep
Or stand six feet apart—
Clutch your heart,
Adjust your face mask—
Memorial Day is very
Different this year—
COVID deaths surpassed
War dead in weeks—
Body bags stacked
In corridors, backs of trucks,
Hastily bulldozed graves—
Never such a death storm
Since World War Two—
Casualties in Korea, Vietnam, Iraq,
Afghanistan topped in three months—
Shouldn't we fly
The flags at half-mast—

Display gold stars in the windows
Of those so suddenly lost?
Obits jammed into newspapers—
So many lives snuffed out
Like candles at a nursing home
Birthday party—
Can you count them all—
Blazing in their 20s, 30s, 40s,
50s, 60s, 70s—
Virus sweeping through
Veterans' homes
Like silent machine-gun fire—
May Day, May Day!
The high flying life is crashing—
Flyovers by war planes
Won't raise the dead, the dying—

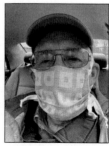

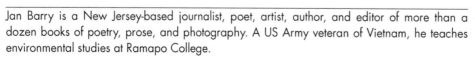

Jan Barry is a New Jersey-based journalist, poet, artist, author, and editor of more than a dozen books of poetry, prose, and photography. A US Army veteran of Vietnam, he teaches environmental studies at Ramapo College.

April Energy 2020

Kathleen Waldron

Longer days with promising warm breezes
Sweet aroma of earth and blossoms
Soft colors—green white pink
Lazy nods of daffodils.
As a child I picked violets near the woods
In April with my friends on Good Friday.
We kept the "Silence" as we picked them
Because Jesus was on the cross.
We ran through the orchards under cherry trees.
I loved April energy.
Later I found lilac bushes growing in Manhattan
In Inwood Hill Park among the trees in the woods.
Someone had a house here a long time ago.
I picked sprigs of lilacs to bring them home
As April became glorious May.
This year I see nothing and
I smell no sweet lilacs.
I sit still, frozen like winter's plaything,
All my energy drained by his passing.
He was tortured by the vicious virus.
My friend was taken just as April's energy burst forth.
I must put lilacs on his grave.
Ventilator and dialysis, completely alone

He had no chance
A vigorous man in good health
Who would think—
One day full of life, ten days later—gone.
We had laughed so much together
And he loved our conversations as I did.
Our families, our work, poetry, our fears,
Childhood memories of our church
He always wanted to be a priest
But the church said no!
He left the church long ago and I prayed
For his conversion but never told him.
He was a wonderful son to his mother
Caring for her during her long last illness.
I dreamed that Mary the Mother of us all
Has shown him now God's mercy and
Welcomed him into the garden
Where April is eternal and
He will be surrounded forever by cherry blossoms and lilacs.

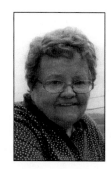

Kathleen Waldron enjoys writing with various groups in the Hudson Valley. Though she thinks about writing a memoir, it appears her gift may be poetry.

HIDDEN EFFECTS

Living in "Corona City" challenged us in unexpected ways. Quarantine and isolation were medically necessary, but they also destroyed important social resources for many who depended on them. The elderly could not receive visitors. Recovering addicts could not attend support gatherings. Those with mental illness couldn't see their therapists. On the other hand, we embraced technology and devised new ways to bring people together online.

VOICES FROM AN EPICENTER
Page 79

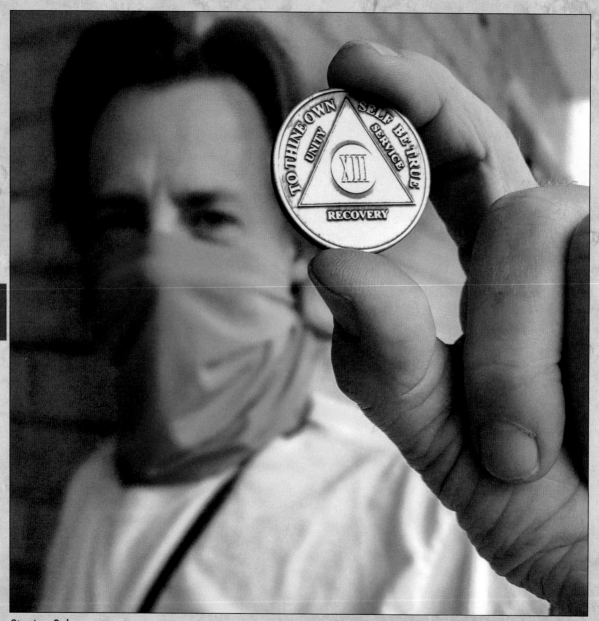

Staying Sober
Maintaining one's sobriety during COVID-19 has been challenging for many as AA meetings are closed. I did not want to miss out on getting my thirteen-year sober anniversary coin so I asked a friend to present it to me at her place on the Upper West Side in Manhattan, May 17, 2020 (Photo by Christopher Monroe)

The Other Epidemic

Keaton Douglas

June 10, 2020

"Hey, u good? Haven't heard from you for a while," I texted Sean, a member of my "team."

As director of a ministry that helps pull people out of the opioid crisis, I checked in with all my teammates regularly, especially during the COVID-19 pandemic when we couldn't see each other. My "teammates" are men and women in the early stages of recovery who'd come through our program and now volunteer their time and talents to help others out of the abyss of addiction. In a 12-step program, they'd be putting step 12—"carrying the message"—into place.

Sean replied several hours later: "I'm okay. At least I'm working."

Not the expected response. Sean was a veritable cheerleader for those in recovery. Just over two years clean from every drug known to mankind, he'd found a real role leading Alcoholics Anonymous (AA) and Narcotics Anonymous (NA) meetings throughout northern New Jersey. He'd been such a force of positivity for others that I often reminded him to make room for "Sean time," lest his own recovery be forgotten.

I texted him back: "That doesn't sound like you. Everything ok? LMK."

When I received no answer, I became concerned. The next morning I heard that Jayda, Sean's friend from high school, had found him unresponsive from an overdose of fentanyl-laced heroin. She administered CPR. The paramedics administered three doses of NARCAN, the drug that reverses opioid overdoses. Jayda and Sean had gotten reacquainted several years earlier after Sean's wife died of an overdose. Even though she wasn't in recovery, Jayda had a real sense of Sean's goodness and related to him in a way that put him at ease.

Sean was rushed to the hospital and remained there in a medically induced coma for weeks. He had "nodded out," as heroin addicts do, and fallen on his own arm. His arms already looked like decorative gourds you'd put out at Thanksgiving—lumpy and bumpy from the aftermath of the many explosions his skin had endured while injecting cocaine. This time he'd cut off the circulation long enough to make saving the arm a worry. He'd also sent himself into acute renal failure. The prognosis for a full recovery was, and remains, slight, though his weakened body continues to fight.

Sean and many others in recovery are the collateral damage of the COVID-19 crisis. Worldwide, people have been affected by the anxiety and depression of self-exile and quarantine—those in recovery, or seeking to be, all the more so. Anxiety, depression, and isolation are hallmarks of any addicted lifestyle. That's why an individual seeking recovery must connect with a community.

Like families, communities are a building block of our society. They help define us, and in them we find collective solutions to problems. With the pandemic came the suspension of the communities found in the fellowship meetings of AA and NA and the like.

Many online video conferences were offered, but many found those platforms to be impersonal interfaces, a perverse "Hollywood Squares" that in no way took the place of in-person fellowship. They missed the handshake of welcome followed by a hot cup of coffee and an invitation to share the day's heartaches and hopes. For some, videoconferencing was not even available because they didn't have the means to own the correct device or weren't savvy enough to understand the technology.

For those suffering from substance use disorders, the pandemic exacerbated the drug and alcohol crisis that already existed. Statistics provided by NJCares.gov, a dashboard of opioid-related data, shows suspected drug- and alcohol-related deaths in New Jersey alone, through April 2020, are up 30 percent from the same time last year.

For a nation that sees more than seventy thousand people die from drug overdoses annually, a 30 percent increase would be a staggering number—and one that doesn't even take into account those individuals who are still using or who turned to drugs and alcohol to assuage the fear and anxiety that COVID-19 created.

As the pandemic passes, let us not forget those who survived the virus but are victims of the loneliness it left in its wake.

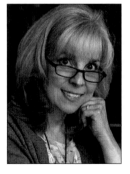

Keaton Douglas is executive director of the iTHIRST Initiative, a mission of the Missionary Servants of the Most Holy Trinity, an international community of Catholic priests and brothers serving the poor and abandoned in thirty-nine missions on two continents. The iTHIRST Initiative empowers faith communities to become a resource for those suffering from addictions and their families. For more information, visit www.iTHIRSTinitiative.org

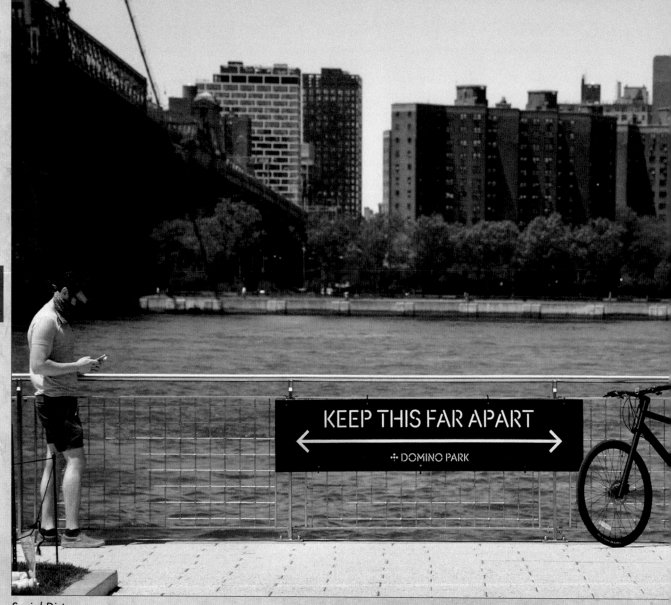

Social Distance
Domino Park, Williamsburg, Brooklyn, New York, May 30, 2020
(Photo by Emma Tager)

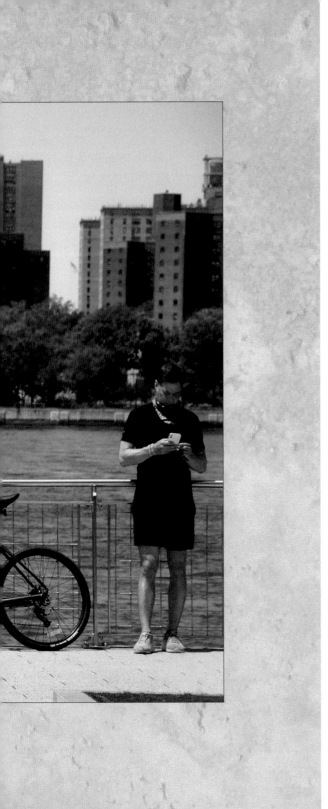

Loneliness of the Elderly

Nancy Mahoney-Rajs

April 14, 2020

Entering through the chapel door, I leave behind the bright sunny day. On the steps to the basement I take my place on the blue taped line. We all stand our distance from each other—nurses, certified nursing assistants, administrators, kitchen staff, several therapists, and me, the dietitian. Masked, gloved, and shielded, we await our quick check overs and disinfectant procedures before entering the New Jersey assisted living facility where we work.

This is our new normal though there's nothing normal about residents living behind their doors, so grateful to see a human face when meals are delivered to their rooms. Nor is there anything normal about the kisses and birthday greetings they receive through a window as their family members socially distance from each other on the front lawn. Their loved ones wear nylon gloves stretched over each hand. Their masks are glued to their faces, and their glasses fog over from their taken breaths. What should have been a joyful visit is laden with these obstacles.

The days are now saturated with longing. Residents pine for a touch or to see another's smile. The sound of loud televisions fills the corridors and rushes through the gaps around doors. Wild turkeys peck at the glass windows as if to ask why their friends inside are not filling their tin feeding dish.

Coworkers, scared and exhausted, feel a sorrowful wrenching as another resident is transported to the hospital. Although our questions are unspoken, we ponder whether the resident will return to us. If they do come back, we wonder, what scars of memory loss or new health conditions will be permanent?

As incomprehensible as it sounds, there are some lucky deaths in the era of COVID-19. The lucky ones are folks at the end of their life, dying from natural causes, because their family is allowed to be present. Covered with safety gear, these family members are allowed to sit at the bedside, weeping, holding hands, and stroking the hair of their loved one, while so many others with the virus slip into the darkness, empty-handed and alone.

According to reports released today, almost 40 percent of coronavirus deaths in New Jersey were residents at nursing facilities. Meanwhile, in New York, "only" twenty-two hundred came from nursing homes. Only? Each one of them died alone, without a loved one by their side. They were only a mother, only a father, only a sibling, only a grandparent, only an aunt, only an uncle, only a friend, only a neighbor.

As with all passing disasters, we will eventually emerge from this one, timidly at first and older in our bodies and our souls. As time goes by, the intensity will lessen when we can once again embrace family, whisper to a friend, nuzzle grandchildren, and sit together in a room sharing stories.

Of course, though, there will be one day a year when we lower our flags and honor those lost. Like the virus, however, even this act of respect will eventually become just a memory.

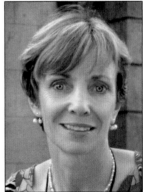

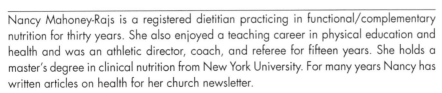

Nancy Mahoney-Rajs is a registered dietitian practicing in functional/complementary nutrition for thirty years. She also enjoyed a teaching career in physical education and health and was an athletic director, coach, and referee for fifteen years. She holds a master's degree in clinical nutrition from New York University. For many years Nancy has written articles on health for her church newsletter.

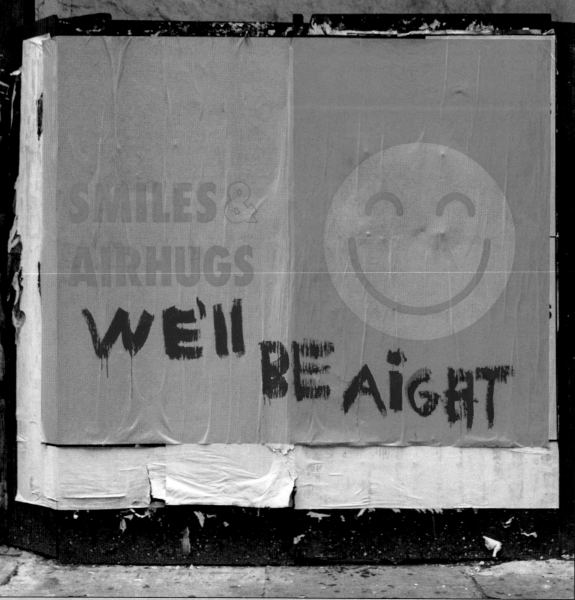

Hopeful Sign
Manhattan, April 10, 2020 (Photo by Walter Wlodarczyk)

Turning to Virtual Therapy

Derk Replogle

work with people for whom isolation can be toxic, sometimes deadly—those struggling with substance use and mental health disorders. In early March I had many all-consuming discussions with clients about COVID-19. I refocused therapy on the importance of self-care and debunked whatever rumors were swirling at the time. I developed a mantra with everyone: "Wash your hands, wear a mask, get sleep. It's just like the flu. We are all going to be fine."

Of course I wasn't so certain we'd be fine, but I said it anyway.

On March 19, 2020 I conducted my last physical group session. Everybody was anxious but dealing well. We discussed the fact that the group would likely be closing, maybe for a few weeks at most.

"When will we be able to come back?" one client asked.

"You can't close," another said. "I need this group."

I reassured them we'd figure everything out. And so I did, setting the stage for a new telehealth counseling group though I had no concept how to create one.

The following week, at the governor's behest, I began working from home. At first everyone—staff and clients—was inexperienced with telehealth. Few of the insurance companies my nonprofit deals with even pay for telehealth services. But we plunged in. Quickly picking a few accessible platforms such as Doxy.me and Zoom, we struggled our way through the learning curve. Technological roadblocks and inexperience plagued staff and clients alike, but we forged ahead. All the players reported feeling the same dominant emotion—anxiety.

I recommended that my clients take a media break. The information highway at the time was flooded with conflicting and anxiety-provoking information. I encouraged them to get their information only from the CDC website. This helped them focus and eased anxiety.

I worried a great deal about my clients. Though not impossible, it's difficult to heal when isolated. We humans are social creatures. My last experience working under duress came after Hurricane Sandy struck New Jersey in 2012. A trend held true in both situations: People used to isolation, either by choice or circumstance, were fine. Withdrawing from society even made some happy.

For others, though, sheltering in place was the first real isolation they'd ever experienced—and addiction is a disease of isolation. One woman I'll call Susan was celebrating her second year of sobriety. Suddenly, she was unable to visit her elderly sponsor, her siblings, and even her own children because they worked in healthcare. She was told the quarantine was "for your own good." But she shared that alone, without her family and supports, and with the fear of illness, she was isolated with her own inner demons again. They brought back the urge to drink stronger than ever.

And there were relapses, which did not surprise me or my colleagues. No one learns to ride a bicycle on the first attempt. Relapse is married to recovery. Without statistics, I will say relapse was higher during the early and middle stages of the pandemic. After self-help meetings and other support groups brought their services online, things shifted. People had a new way to be together. Anxiety gradually eased as people reconnected, engaged in active therapy, and shared with their peers. The workers who migrated services online are unsung heroes of this coronavirus event.

Simultaneously, telehealth brought new challenges, such as managing interruptions by children and homelife. Not all people have the luxury of privacy. One of my clients I'll call Mary was isolated at home with her seven children, ages two to seventeen. While on the phone with me, she was rarely able to complete a single thought without being interrupted.

The deeper we went into the pandemic, the more fear, ongoing uncertainty, and grief over lost family and friends crept into sessions and groups. So did partisan politics. It's difficult to create an atmosphere where clients can vent but not trample on other members with differing political viewpoints. Eventually, the routine of quarantine and isolation gave way to boredom and drudgery. Clients wanted to return to face-to-face sessions. So did I. Nuances, behavioral cues, and paralanguage are difficult to observe during telehealth. Losing them detracts from the clinical picture and interpersonal exchanges.

Through everything, though, my thirty-plus clients endured. They innovated. They created. They asked for help. They helped each other. They became stronger.

As I write this, I recognize we're far from the pandemic's end. For many the trauma will endure for years. That's not what I'll remember, though.

I'll remember the tenacity and resilience of both my clients and peers. We choose whether a crisis will define us or mobilize us into stronger people. Fortunately, I have witnessed the latter.

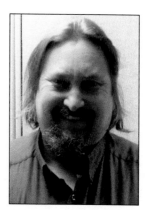

Derk Replogle, MA, LCADC, CCS, is a therapist in a New Jersey nonprofit community mental health and addiction services program. He serves as director of addiction services, supervisor, and team member.

NEW REALITIES

COVID-19 became so pervasive, it changed even the most basic of human experiences—how lovers loved, how mothers gave birth, how we shopped for food, how we protested in the streets, how we went through non-COVID medical events like cancer surgery. The virus revealed something else—social inequities. To some it meant freedom, even leisure. To others, including the unemployed, it brought anxiety and hardship.

VOICES
FROM AN
EPICENTER
Page 93

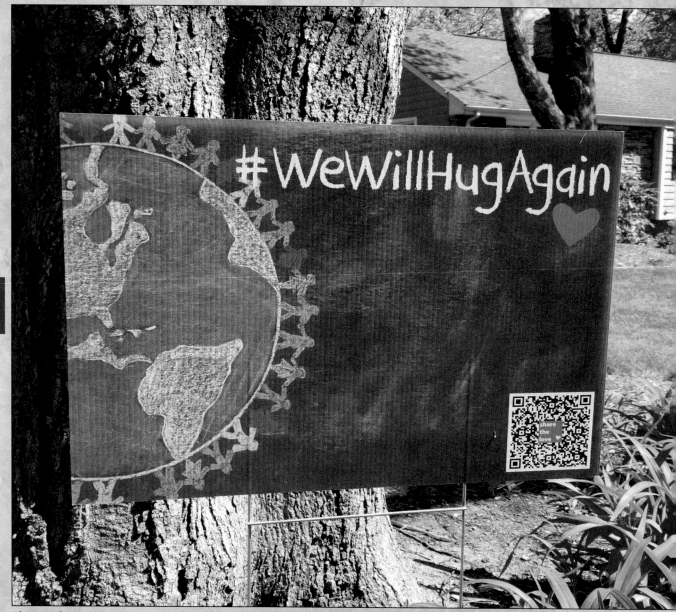

Sharing the Love
This #WeWillHugAgain yard sign, created by a Bethlehem, Pennsylvania printing service,
appears throughout the New York Metro Area, May 2020 (Photo by **Lorraine Ash**)

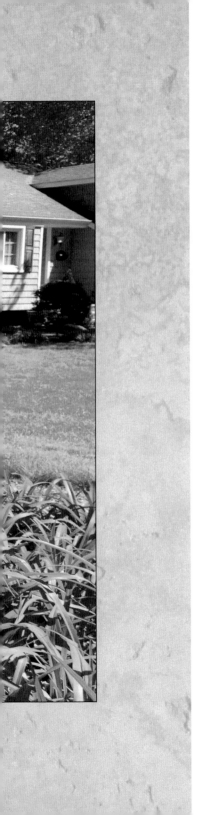

Into His Arms—Or Not

Jean Sheff

May 12, 2020

I hear him as he slides the key into my front door lock. The sound of metal on metal makes my insides lurch, but I swivel my desk chair to face the door. Michael and I have navigated the twenty-five minutes between our homes for four years with a boldness we no longer possess.

When the COVID-19 shelter-in-place orders went into effect, we were each in our own homes.

"Jean, with your autoimmune issues, I'm the worst thing for you," he said. "I couldn't bear it if you got sick."

That wasn't what I wanted to hear. Though I'd been working from home, I'd lost my job because of the virus, just as millions of others had. I was looking at painfully empty days. Yet, he was right. Michael works in the medical field and he'd been seeing patients until our world shuttered closed. Yes, quarantining for two weeks was judicious.

We called one another two or three times a day. We relied on each other to ease the endless hours. Things were grim. New cautions were issued daily. The rules changed by the hour. If you dared to go outside, you had best suit up like an astronaut walking on the moon. We got skittish and held off getting together for another week, then another. People we knew were getting sick. His aunt and uncle, who lived in a local senior center, were whisked off to a hospital. Five days later they were both dead. With funerals banned, we couldn't gather to find comfort. Everyone cried at home alone.

Before we knew it, another several weeks passed. We kept flip-flopping on when to break the quarantine. Where was my bravery? I felt shallow. One night I invited him to dinner for the following day. He called early the next morning. His throat was sore, he said, and his eyes were watering. We cancelled. Paranoia had found a home. A cough felt fatal. I vacillated between feeling ridiculous and not cautious enough. The separation was getting painful. We consulted doctors, friends, and family. No one could reassure us. No one knows what safe is anymore. To get together, we'd have to just take our chances.

So here we are. He's arriving for dinner, and I'm jumpy. He creaks the door open, as if he's afraid, too. I stand. We look at each other. We try to smile. He extends his hand, offering me a dozen ruby roses cradled in cellophane. I want this scene to be different. It should evoke the iconic 1945 Eisenstaedt photo of an impassioned sailor kissing a nurse in Times Square at the end of World War II. Or if not that, then why not the scene in countless films and a legion of novels—two amorous people huddled tightly together as the bombs drop around them?

But in this time of COVID-19, touching is dangerous. I try to will the dread away. Yet fear is insidious. It creeps into every chink in the foundation of my soul. I step forward and take the roses, then open my arms to him. We hug. It feels like there's a saguaro cactus wedged between our chests. It hurts. I turn my head into his shoulder and grab him tighter. For the rest of the evening we're careful with each other. After dinner we watch some television and relax enough to hold hands. He rises to leave and we hug again, but we don't kiss.

Being deprived of touch feels cruel. In so many ways it sustains me. I miss human contact, from a dear one's hug to a friendly handshake to a lover's embrace. With masks shielding us from one another, I even miss seeing the smiles of people I don't know. But this is the new human condition.

Later, I get into bed and cocoon myself in the covers. I'm lonelier now than at any time during the seven weeks we spent apart. I turn over, wondering how we'll come together again. Still, we're just two. How will everyone in this country, in this world, ever come together again?

I challenge myself: *if I weren't thinking so much about this, what would I be feeling?* I can't go there. I shut down. An anthem enshrines this pandemic— "We're in This Together." Maybe that's because, as in birth and death, the truth is, we're in this alone.

Jean Sheff holds a BFA from Adelphi University. She is an award-winning, New York-based writer and editor. Jean is devoted to her daughter, Juliana, and enjoys teaching Pilates.

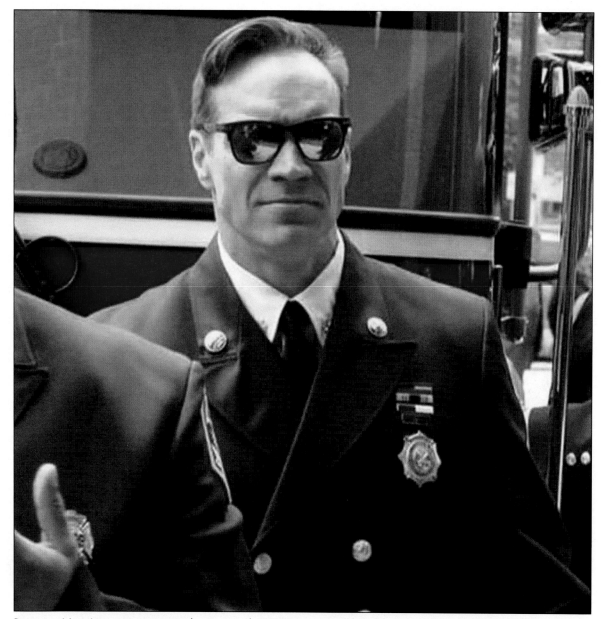

Paterson, New Jersey was a city under siege with COVID cases and their first responders answered the call
(Photo Courtesy of Vincent T. Marchese)

Making Masks

Sue Farrar Dinetz

March 10

My mask making started about March 10, 2020, several weeks before most realized critical personal protective equipment (PPE) was in short supply. When the crisis began my son Cameron Gardner, a deputy chief with the Paterson Fire Department, was immediately reassigned as coordinator of the Office of Emergency Management. Paterson was a war zone, COVID was rampant, everyone was desperate for PPE, and he was right in the thick of it all. Calls were coming in from rehabs, shelters, and group homes, all asking for help as their staffs navigated the pandemic. In all his years as a firefighter, this was the first time I saw him look concerned—very concerned.

This was the moment I decided to help. Despite a vague recollection from my limited religious instruction that God didn't make deals with people, I offered Him a bargain: if He would protect my son from contracting COVID, I would make masks for anyone who needed them for as long as they needed them.

I've made more than twelve hundred masks and never charged anyone a penny—not even for postage, despite my husband's protestations. In return,

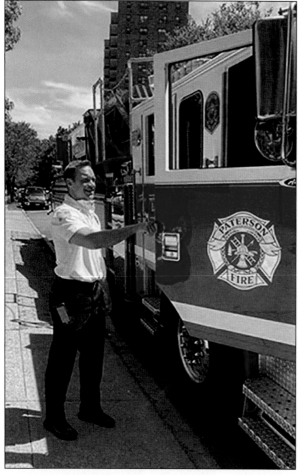

Deputy Chief Gardner inspects the apparatus
(Photo by Sue Farrar Dinetz)

I received countless blessings and a soul refueled on high test. And this much has been reaffirmed: there are far more good people in the world than not.

Early on, I complained on Facebook that my fifty-year-old Singer was giving me a hard time. I kept hitting my finger on a piece of jagged metal until it became infected. A stranger saw my post and offered to give me a brand new, unused Singer sewing machine that her father had given to her mother and her mother had given to her. Though forty years old, it had never been out of the box. How perfect! No learning curve. All she asked was that I continue sewing masks.

Soon it became apparent that the green produce twist ties I'd been stealing from the supermarket for my masks (a small sin in the context of a much bigger picture) weren't strong enough to create a tight-fitting seal by the bridge of the nose. I read somewhere that Sheet Metal Workers Local 22 out of Cranford, New Jersey, made metal nose clips designed to give masks a snug fit. I reached out to the union. The very next day a driver came to my house with one hundred metal clips! Tom Fischbach, the union's president, wrote me a letter offering me as many clips as needed, free of charge.

The Company Store donated fabric. Brother donated thirty sewing machines to what was then a sewing group because, yes, about forty local people offered to help with the effort. We even created a Facebook group, NJ Masks, to coordinate our efforts. Volunteers who couldn't sew performed other tasks: they cut fabric, delivered supplies, and picked up finished masks.

Those who received free masks sent notes of gratitude with gift cards or cash while others sent me pieces of their heart. One woman asked for two masks—one for her, one for her daughter. I mailed them out, as I had so many others. She replied with this touching note accompanied by a painting she'd made for me:

Thank you for your exceptional kindness and willingness to make masks for a complete stranger. I reached out to you and you responded without hesitation. Please enjoy this painting I made for you. I call it "Farrar's Iris," inspired by your beautiful spirit.

Jan Cornero

All I did was sew masks. I neither expected nor wanted anything in return because, after all, I'd made an important deal with the man upstairs. I was merely keeping up my end of the bargain. God certainly kept up His end as well and multiplied the blessings a hundredfold.

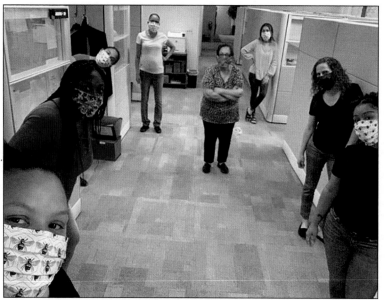

Staff at Lifeline OB/GYN model their handmade masks
(Courtesy of Felicita Bermudez)

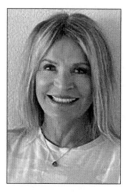

Sue Farrar Dinetz is a semiretired dilettante. She attended Bergen Community College for nursing, The Finishing School in New York for decorative wall finishes, and County College of Morris, where she earned her certification in phlebotomy. Most recently, she worked at a COVID-19 test site performing nasal swabs and completed the Johns Hopkins University course in contact tracing. She lives in Morris Plains, New Jersey. www.NJMasks.com

Birth in the Time of Corona

Kara Naegely

April 2020

"I'm gonna throw up."

"That's just the morphine. We just put the anti-nausea medication in your IV now. It should kick in soon. You'll be alright."

You can't vomit all over this operating room—it's sterile. They'll probably make you start all over again. You don't want another spinal tap. No ... I want my mom.

"I'm definitely going to throw up." I barely get the words out before I gag.

I feel someone put a bag in my hand and pull it up to my face. *How am I going to do this? I'm flat on my back with zero feeling from my breasts down. I can't sit up. I can't roll over. My own body is useless to me. Here we go.* I heave and vomit into the tiny airplane barf bag. The majority of mucousy regurgitation goes all over the side of my face and into my hair.

"Thank you." I cough and sheepishly add, "I'm sorry."

"Here she is!" I feel a presence at my right shoulder. "Hi, babe." My wife is with me now. *Thank God.*

"I threw up," I say, flatly.

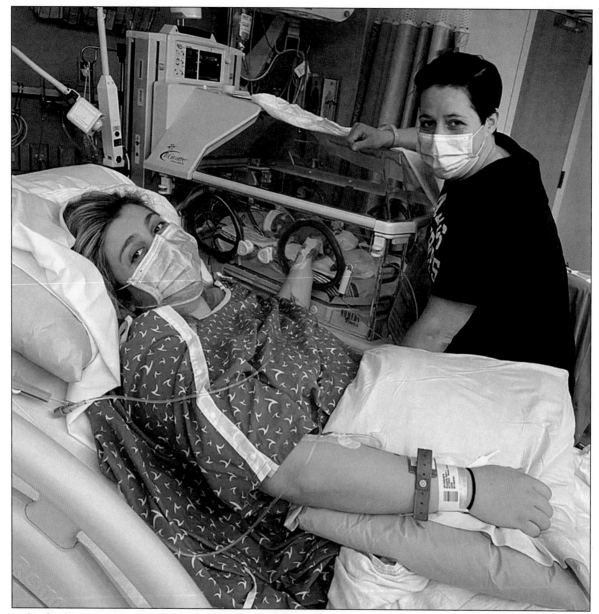

Right after her C-section, Kara Naegely visits her daughter, Kellyn, in the Neonatal Intensive Care Unit, as her wife, Liz Sisca, comforts them both, April, 2020 (Courtesy of Kara Naegely)

I begin to feel my body being jerked. It shakes as the surgeons cut into each layer of fat and muscle. I keep my eyes closed and focus only on my breathing and the stroke of Liz's hand on my head. Then I hear her little voice, *Ehh ehh.* She isn't crying. Rather, she sounds like someone awakened from a nap too soon—unpleasantly surprised to see it's daytime and people are expecting her to be social.

"She's perfect!" Liz cries. She kisses my forehead.

Her little head peeks over the curtain and I see my daughter's face for the first time. I'm already in love. The nurses clean her up and bring her over to say hello to her mamas. She gives us a quick "kiss" through our masks before she's taken away.

Once I've been sewn up and my doctor graciously washes the vomit out of my hair, I am wheeled back to my room for recovery—without my baby. My newborn baby girl will be

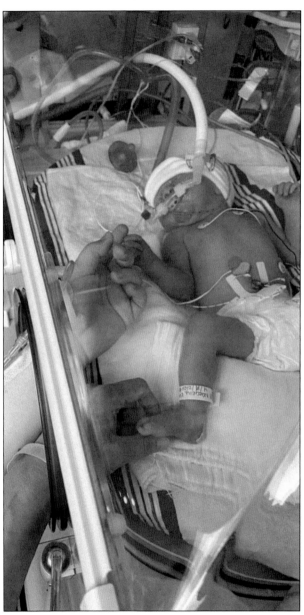

Kellyn gets plenty of support from her mothers in the NICU, April, 2020 (Courtesy of Kara Naegely)

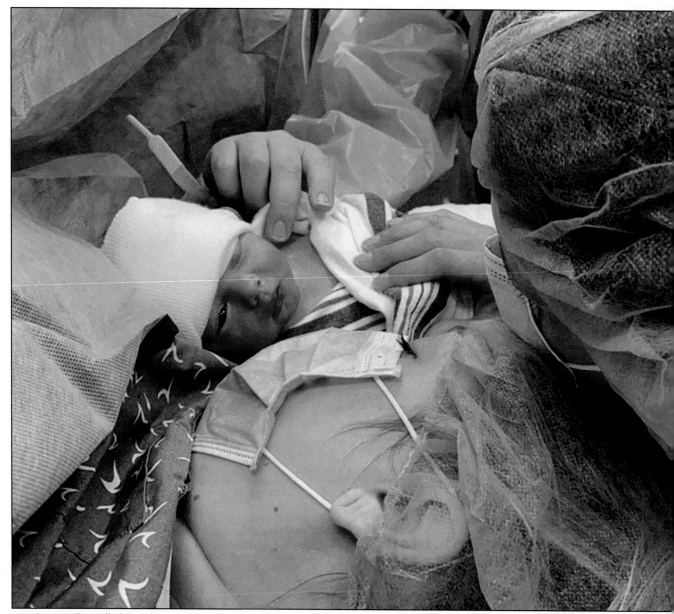

Newborn Kellyn, all cleaned up, meets her mothers in the operating room, April, 2020 (Courtesy of Kara Naegely)

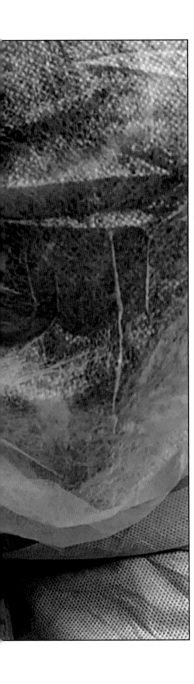

staying in the NICU. Liz and I will be permitted to visit one at a time, once a day, for two hours. I can hear my heart breaking.

"Can we at least get her in there to see the baby today?" Liz begs the nurses. "This isn't right. Please."

"Come on, let's go," I hear someone say. Two nurses unlock the wheels on my bed, grab my IVs, and roll me down to the NICU. There she is—my little Kellyn. I hold her hand through the opening in the incubator as I survey the tubes and wires taped all over her five-pound body. *We made it.*

We spend the rest of the day in our room calling our parents, family, and closest friends to let them know the delivery was a success and that baby and mom are fine. There is no pomp and circumstance, no flowers or balloons, no welcoming committee for Kellyn. We are alone. The only visitors we have are the nurses who routinely check my vitals, refill my magnesium drip, empty my urine drainage bag, draw my blood, and take both our temperatures to ensure neither of us has a fever.

The nurses become our adopted friends and bring us extra food and snacks. We weren't prepared.

"I was only here for extra lab work Saturday morning," I tell the nurses. "We weren't expecting to be here so long."

The doctors wanted to monitor me for preeclampsia and HELLP. By Saturday afternoon, I was admitted. By early Saturday evening, I was being scheduled for a Sunday morning C-section. Once I was admitted, Liz couldn't leave the hospital. If she had, she would not have been able to return.

The next day Liz pushes me in my wheelchair and takes me to hold Kellyn for the first time.

"Neither of us has the virus," Liz says. "This is our first child. We absolutely can't come in together?" I hear the desperation in her voice. I have been surprisingly good at maintaining my composure throughout the whole ordeal.

"No," we are told, due to "policy."

We alternate our visits with Kellyn. For the next three days one of us dons a mask and visits while the other watches the interaction via webcam from my room. We are discharged on Wednesday without our baby. Still unable to eat without the assistance of a feeding tube, she has to remain in the care of the NICU. We cry the whole ride home, every cell in our bodies revolting against leaving our child behind.

The alternating visits continue until we bring Kellyn home the following Saturday afternoon. After two years of fertility treatments, five IUIs, two IVFs, tens of thousands of dollars, preeclampsia, HELLP, an emergency C-section six weeks early, and a pandemic, I am finally able to kiss my daughter's head, lips to skin. No mask.

She sees my face for the first time in her short, dramatic life and she smiles.

Kara Naegely is an animal lover, mental health advocate, artist, and bookworm. She lives in New Jersey with her wife and two children—one human, one Maltese. Kara currently works in patient assistance but aspires to write full-time.

Shopping, an Odyssey

William J. Burrows

April 7, 2020

"Sorry, Love, you're the kids' crisis school teacher today."

Loretta groans as she stretches before getting out of bed.

"Oh yeah, today's the day my knight in shining armor does battle for the family," she says.

"I'm just doing the shopping," I reply.

"Yes, but you're the one taking risks. I'm just glad you decided to only do this once every three weeks."

"I've forgotten my Alexa password," I tell her, "so I couldn't retrieve the shopping list."

"Don't worry, I'll text it," Loretta answers. "Do you have Mom's list?"

"Yep, plus my mask, plastic gloves, and a couple of bottles of water."

"Great, now go before you miss the senior opening hours."

I leave home at 8:25 a.m. I pull into the Costco car park at 8:55 a.m. The queue to get in is already three times the length of the building. A policeman leans on a police car parked outside the front doors. *We need a police presence to go shopping?*

I put on my mask and gloves and grab my bags. As I approach the queue's end, a staff member stops me and wipes the handle of my shopping wagon with a disinfectant cloth. The policeman walks towards the lines.

"Those age sixty and over, queue to the right," he shouts. "Under sixty, to the left." *There are younger people already queuing to go in at 10 a.m.?*

Less than ten minutes later, I find myself inside the store.

"Please maintain social distancing," a staff member calls out. Everyone seems to be doing their best to comply.

This is the easy shop—nothing for Mom here, just what's on Loretta's list times three! Only one brand of toilet rolls are in stock. There are no kitchen towels or hand sanitizers. I miss the tasting stations, but that means I get to the centralized register queue reasonably quickly. Each shopper is standing on a six-foot marker on the floor.

"Please stay behind the line until the cashier calls you forward," says a masked staff member as she points to a marker behind a register to my right. The cashier calls me forward and scans my membership card while I hold it. As she scans my items behind her plexiglass barrier, I notice her fingernails have perforated her plastic gloves. Frantically, I try to keep up as I bag my own groceries.

At the exit someone behind a protective screen checks my receipt and waves me on—no marking receipts these days.

Next I go to Walmart and start my mother-in-law's shopping. The queue to get into the store seems shorter. Yet it's a full fifteen minutes before I get in. Here I'm only shopping for one, but at eighty-six, Mom has acquired some specific tastes. *Hungry-man chicken meals with mashed potato and vegetables. Okay, fried or roast chicken? Mixed vegetables or green beans? Hmm, there's only one type, but it's patties, I'm sure she said she doesn't like patties.*

The deli counter is closed. There are arrows on the floor, but no one seems to notice, or if they do, they aren't paying attention. Whole aisles are stripped bare; there are no pasta or paper products, only one brand of flour. I finish shopping, having found no more than about half the items on Mom's list.

I drive to ShopRite, where there is no queue outside. I find alternatives for everything on her list except BBQ Shake 'n Bake. I pray Mom will understand and like everything I've gotten her.

I arrive at Mom's condo and sign in. I place the pen in the provided box so it can be disinfected later. Mom meets me at her door with her mask on.

"Don't forget to disinfect everything before you put it away," I tell her. We bump elbows as I leave.

■

"Hi, Love, I'm home," I shout as I open the front door.

"Oh, great," she replies. "I'll grab my gloves and the disinfectant spray."

"It could take awhile," I say. "There's a lot!"

At 3:10 p.m. I collapse on the sofa, hugging a hot cup of coffee. All the boxes have been wiped, the fruit washed. Everything is away. Loretta settles in beside me.

"Nearly seven hours," she says, "and Mom wonders why you only want to do this once every three weeks!"

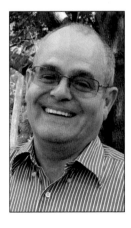

William J. Burrows is a somewhat reclusive writer, devoted father, and shy missionary. He is on a crusade to use his life experiences as a means to help others.

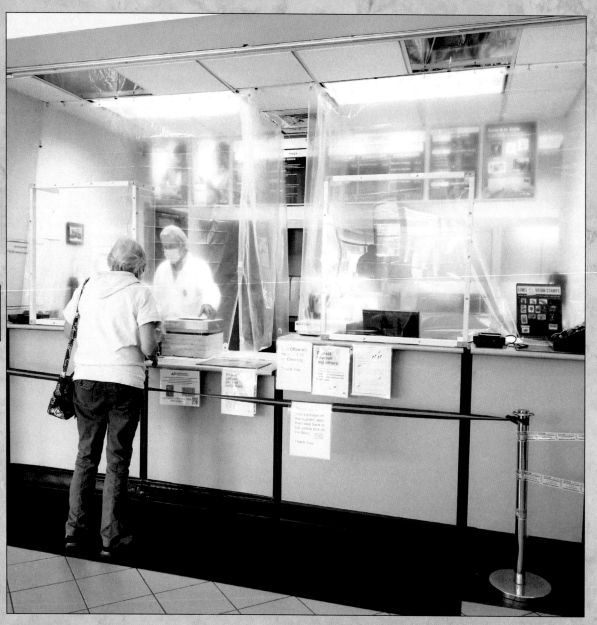

Delivering Safety
A local post office in Bergen County, New Jersey pulls out all the stops to protect its employees and patrons and keep packages moving, May 2020 (Photo by Lorraine Ash)

Cancer Is Enough

Darcey Gohring

A month before COVID-19 hit New Jersey, I was a busy forty-six-year-old mother, driving two active teenagers from game to game. I worked on freelance writing jobs and volunteered for local organizations. An avid runner, I averaged fifteen to twenty miles a week. I was the kind of person most people would describe as "healthy as a horse." No red flags on my medical radar. No genetic history of anything unusual, either. In fact, in the past fifteen years, I'd never been to a doctor for anything more than a once-a-year physical and maybe a sinus infection.

Just like most other people in the New York/New Jersey area, I watched the initial news reports about coronavirus, thinking it was scary but would be nothing more than an inconvenience for a couple of weeks.

When schools closed in mid-March, my heart broke for the victims, but I appreciated the family time we were getting together—playing board games, working on puzzles, and baking cookies.

By April, as the number of cases began to explode in our region, I worried about my husband, who has asthma, my mother, and other family members I saw as potentially more vulnerable. Never once did I worry about me. Instead

I assigned myself the supermarket shopper, sending texts to anyone who I thought might need groceries and dropping bags of food on their porches.

And then one night as I sat on the couch mindlessly watching television, everything changed. As I adjusted my sports bra, my fingers grazed something the size of a large pea under the soft squishy skin of my breast. I could move it under the surface. What I knew most was, it wasn't supposed to be there. And just like that, I was the vulnerable one.

After a frantic late-night email, my doctor arranged to see me the next morning. Days later, a mammogram, biopsy, and ultrasound confirmed the mass was cancer. Those initial doctor and hospital visits were scarier than anything I'd ever done. Each time, I went alone. Each time, I worried that in addition to maybe having cancer, I might also expose myself to getting the coronavirus.

And as I navigated the unchartered waters of my first real medical crisis, what I resented most was not the diagnosis itself, but all the things that would be different if it weren't for COVID-19. In weak moments they played in my mind, reminding me how much easier even this experience would be if things were just back to normal.

I'd have someone to accompany me in waiting rooms instead of sitting next to taped-off empty chairs with signs attached: "Maintain six feet of separation." I wouldn't have to go to consultations alone, trying my best to hold it together and retain all the information the doctors threw at me.

The day of my surgery, my husband and I arrived at the hospital, greeted outside by a police officer.

"Patients only, no visitors," he reminded us.

As we said goodbye, me sobbing and clinging to my husband for a few last minutes, my mind flooded with worries. *What if something goes wrong? What if*

I get the virus today? Why do I have to do this all alone? One last squeeze and I forced myself to walk inside, swallowing my tears. Hours later, I awakened from surgery surrounded by strangers outfitted in so many masks and face shields that, even with all their kindness, I would never know any of them on the street.

Back home I recuperated in quarantined isolation, my only lifeline to family and friends coming in texts, emails, or phone calls. A few in-person visits were held outside, with friends strategically positioned. They felt like reminders of just how much I could use a hug. And still I thought that the surgery was the hard part, that the rest was going to be easier. *I'm "lucky,"* I thought. *I "only" have to do radiation, not chemo.*

But nothing prepared me for seemingly endless weeks of treatments. Day after day, I was stopped at the door to have my temperature taken and answered the same two questions: "Have you shown any symptoms of the virus? Have you been in contact with anyone who has tested positive?"

All I could think was, *No, but I have cancer and that's enough, isn't it?*

And then there was the one thing that never went away, that followed me throughout the journey. It found me in doctors' offices, as I lay on metal tables, at CAT scans and MRIs—I didn't let the tears come because you can't *really* cry with a mask on. I've tried.

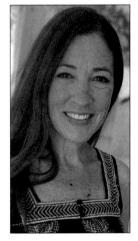

Darcey Gohring is a New Jersey-based freelance writer with more than twenty years of experience. She is the former managing editor of a regional lifestyle magazine and is currently completing her first novel.

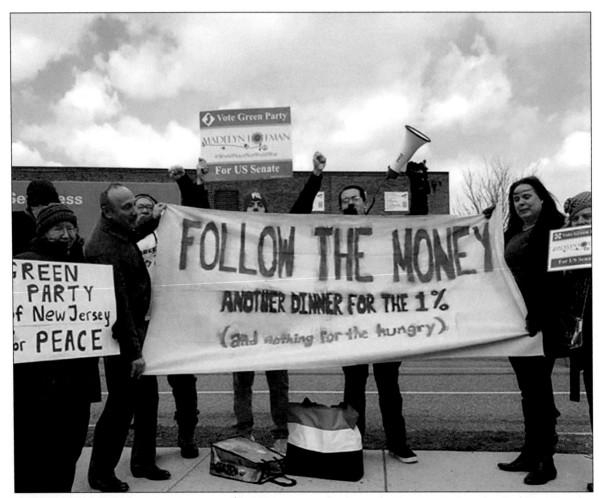

The Green Party of New Jersey protests at a $2,500-per-person fundraiser for Democratic Party leadership at Camden County College, February 29, 2020. Candidate for U.S. Senate, Madelyn Hoffman, is on the far right in her "billionaire outfit" (Courtesy of Heather Warburton)

Protesting, COVID Style

Madelyn Hoffman

Early May 2020

I got a package of face masks in the mail today. I did a little dance, pumped my fist in the air, and then checked myself.

If you'd told me six months ago that getting face masks would be cause for any kind of celebration, I wouldn't have known what to say. I don't like seeing images of people all around the world wearing face masks. It makes me feel like I've somehow landed on another planet. At the same time, when I put one on, it felt strangely liberating.

I haven't stepped inside an enclosed space other than my apartment or car for almost two months. I have pulled up only once to get gas and handed a gas station attendant my credit card. Several times weekly now, I drive to local restaurants to pick up food. Each time I cover my mouth and nose with the fake fur scarf I purchased for the "billionaire" outfit I wore at the last outdoor protest I attended. It took place on the campus of Camden County College in New Jersey on a cold, windy late February afternoon.

Now the place has turned into a COVID-19 testing center. But that afternoon ten members of the Green Party of New Jersey joined my campaign for United

States Senate outside a $2,500-per-person fundraiser for some Democratic Party elites in New Jersey. We charged twenty-five cents for a slice of pizza.

So I would look rich that afternoon, for purposes of the protest, I wore a long black skirt, a black sweater with faux pearls on the front and sleeves, a little gray crocheted hat, two long necklaces of pink stones—and that fake fur scarf. I carried a silver purse over my shoulder. We all unfurled a banner made the night before that read, "FOLLOW THE MONEY—ANOTHER DINNER FOR THE 1% (and nothing for the hungry)."

We were well aware then of what we're seeing now. While money pours into the hands of the political elites, those working for them are often left one or two paychecks away from being hungry and homeless. Little did we know that afternoon how soon we'd witness all our systems fail. Little did we know how our work as activists and Greens would soon become about providing hundreds of meals to senior citizens, immigrant families, families of undocumented workers, families with five children or no children—all needing *someone* to bring them food and necessary supplies.

Until these face masks arrived today, my "billionaire" scarf was all I had to protect myself against the coronavirus and to protect others in case I was an asymptomatic carrier. With a face mask, I feel a little emboldened.

Perhaps I will walk into a supermarket soon and see what's on the shelves. If a mask is required, I will certainly wear one. If it's not, I'll still wear one. It's the least I can do to prevent the spread of a disease so deadly for so many people. I'm sixty-three, just a couple of years away from joining one of the most vulnerable groups—sixty-five and older.

Maybe I'll even take a long walk around my apartment complex. I could use that!

Maybe I'll attend a socially distanced protest in the streets of Newark or Trenton to protest the continued killing of black people while they're jogging or sleeping.

Maybe now I'll step out of the car on a city street instead of only participating in car caravan protests around ICE detention centers. The protests call for all detainees to be released. I can't imagine how terrified these men and women must feel when they can't socially distance. They even have to purchase a bar of soap.

I think about nurses and doctors *still* clamoring for PPE and N95 surgical masks, *still* reporting that they wear the same face mask shift after shift. I saw a protest of nurses in Washington, D.C., honoring eighty-eight nurses who have died from COVID-19.

I also think about the workers at Amazon warehouses, or at meat packing plants, risking exposure rather than lose a $15-per-hour wage with $2-per-hour hazard pay.

Then I see a photograph of Jeff Bezos, Amazon's CEO, posing with his girlfriend in front of the beautiful pond at the Taj Mahal. The headline at the top of the photo reads, "Bezos will soon become a trillionaire." If my face mask were on at that moment, I would have choked into it.

PHOTO: HEATHER WARBURTON

Madelyn Hoffman, a seasoned activist, was director of the Grass Roots Environmental Organization and director of New Jersey Peace Action. She was Ralph Nader's vice-presidential running mate in New Jersey in 1996. The following year she ran for New Jersey governor as a Green. She also ran as a Green for U.S. Senate in 2018, receiving 25,150 votes, and as of this printing is running for the same seat again in 2020.

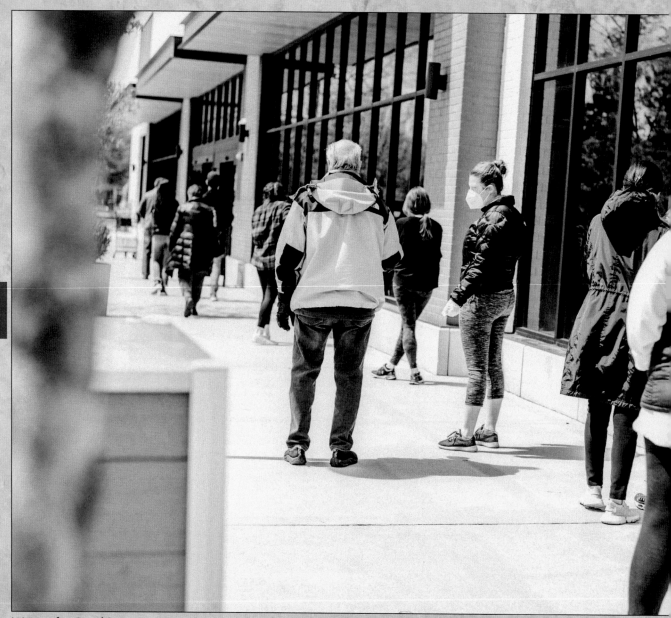

Waiting for Good Buys
Shoppers waiting in line outside of a department store due to
capacity limitations, May 10, 2020 (Photo by Rebecca Osso)

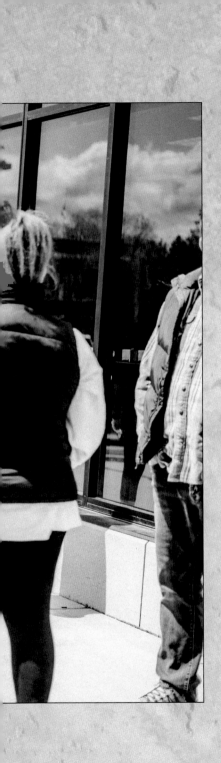

Just Wait

Ali Arje

April 2020

Early on a damp, cloudy April day, I peer ahead of me two hundred feet on the supermarket line and see those at the front. I got here at 7 a.m. to join the senior shoppers. We're allowed entrance at 8 a.m., an hour before the store opens to everyone else. That's because we're the citizens most at risk from COVID-19—the ones with the underlying conditions that the health department talking heads so blithely refer to as "comorbidities." I'm very protective of my underlying conditions. And don't call me comorbid.

Six feet ahead of me is a very elderly woman. Wiry thin with Ivory Snow white hair that matches her face mask, she wraps her raincoat tighter and turns to look behind her. Our gazes meet above our masks. I figure her to be eighty-five, but spry, as they say. Twenty years my senior.

"I had the coronavirus," she tells me across six feet of air. "I didn't know and I gave it to my son. He had to go into the hospital. He was so sick. It's a nightmare, just terrible. People don't know how terrible. They should never know."

With that, she leans hard against a car parked next to the line. I start to lunge toward her to help, then worry I'll be too close and catch myself.

"Why don't you go wait in your car?" I ask. "I'll hold your spot. You can come back when we get close to the door. It's not a problem. Show me where your car is and I'll walk with you."

She shakes her snowy hair.

"Thank you, but I'm okay," she says. "I'm concerned about this gentleman ahead of me. He's really quite old. I'm eighty-eight. He must be up in his nineties. I don't like how unsteady he is. A man that age shouldn't have to stand this long on a line for anything."

She leans hard against the car again. I'm worried. I look six feet behind me and see a woman my age. She's shaking her head.

"They should really have a separate line for people over eighty," she says. "They should just walk them right in the frigging door and not make them wait at all. For God's sake, these people are *elderly*. It's not right."

I ask her to hold my place and I walk to the front of the line, where a twentysomething store employee is fussing with her mask and chatting with the coworker next to her. The line has not moved yet. The door is still shut. It's ten minutes to eight.

"Excuse me," I say, "but I'm halfway down the line and there are two people ahead of me who are quite elderly and standing way too long. Is there some way those who are struggling can be given extra consideration?"

"Well, it's the line for seniors, you know? There's only one line."

"Yes, I see that. But I'm sixty-five and these people ahead of me are much older. The gentleman might be ninety-five. Maybe there's some place they can sit. Can I speak to the manager?"

"The store isn't open yet. And ninety-five is the same as sixty-five. It's all seniors."

Be it youth or ignorance, it takes my breath away. I remind myself that she's an essential worker and she's taking a risk just showing up each day. I walk back to my place in line, thinking of other countries and cultures that value those who have walked the most miles and endured the longest years. I recognize that I don't live in one of those.

The woman behind me asks what I found out. I tell her the young female worker says there's no difference between sixty-five and ninety-five. The woman's eyes narrow.

"You know what you should have told her?" she says. "You should have told her to wait. That's all. Just wait."

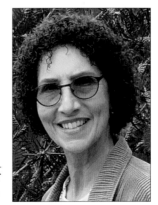

Ali Arje is a journalist, columnist, and blogger. She is currently seeking publication of her children's picture book. Her archived essays can be read at www.OneSaneVoice.com.

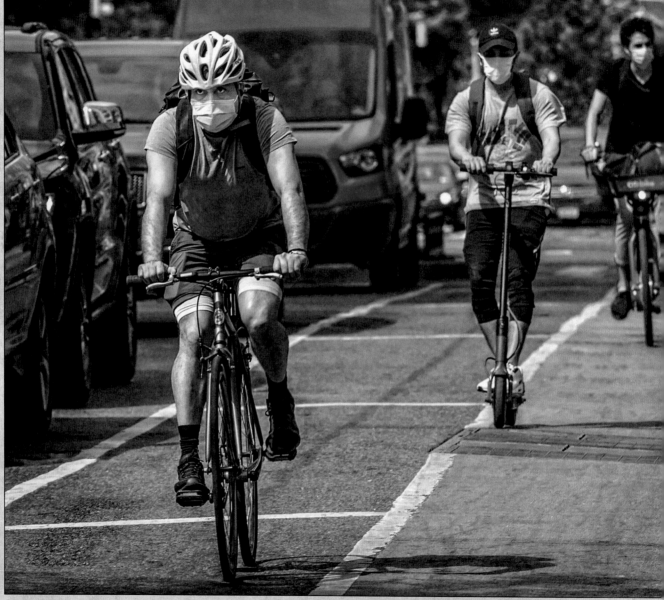

Move On
Riders make their way through New York City streets as people
slowly re-emerge, May 22, 2020 (Photo by Jessica Margo)

The Best and Worst of Times

Ilene Beckerman

In 1859 Charles Dickens wrote in *A Tale of Two Cities*, "It was the best of times, it was the worst of times."

Now, 161 years later, I wonder, *Is this the best of times?*

We're going through a wonderful time, having a pause, a hiatus from the hustle and bustle and responsibilities of everyday life. It's a time when weekdays are like weekends.

It's a time when you never have to look at your watch because time doesn't matter. It's a time when you don't have to go to work or go anywhere.

It's a time when you have time to just think. To get to know who you are now. When you have time to dream all day and sleep as long as you like. You can have breakfast at midnight, dinner at 9 a.m. You can stay in your pajamas all day if you choose. Read. Watch endless entertainment 24-7—movies, music, theater, dance, art, comedy—in your bedroom or living room at no cost (or very low cost), just by turning on your computer, iPad, or TV. You can be creative—start a new hobby.

No gym. No workouts. Take a walk instead. How lucky we are these Corona days.

Wouldn't you call it the best of times?

But what if you had no job, no salary coming in? Couldn't pay the rent or shop for food? What if you couldn't visit with family that wasn't actually living with you? Or have coffee or a beer with friends? What if you were confined to your apartment or house 24-7? What if your kids couldn't go to school? What if when you had to go out to see your doctor or get your meds, you had to wear a mask that covered your nose and mouth? What if you were told never to touch your face? What if you were told to wash your hands every time you touched something?

What if people you knew were dying every day from an invisible enemy? What if someone in your family were next? What if you were next?

Wouldn't you call it the worst of times?

I wonder, *Did Charles Dickens know what the year 2020 would be like?*

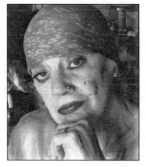

Ilene Beckerman is the author of the best-selling memoir *Love, Loss, and What I Wore*, which was also the inspiration for the off-Broadway hit of the same name. Algonquin Books has published all five of her books. http://lovelossandreallife.com

EDUCATION

School and childcare posed a unique set of challenges. As we grappled with the need to educate our children and keep them and their teachers safe, we faced important questions: How do we teach our kids and stay sane? How do working parents take on the additional role of ensuring lessons are learned? Are rich and poor students affected differently when brick-and-mortar schools close?

VOICES
FROM AN
EPICENTER
Page 127

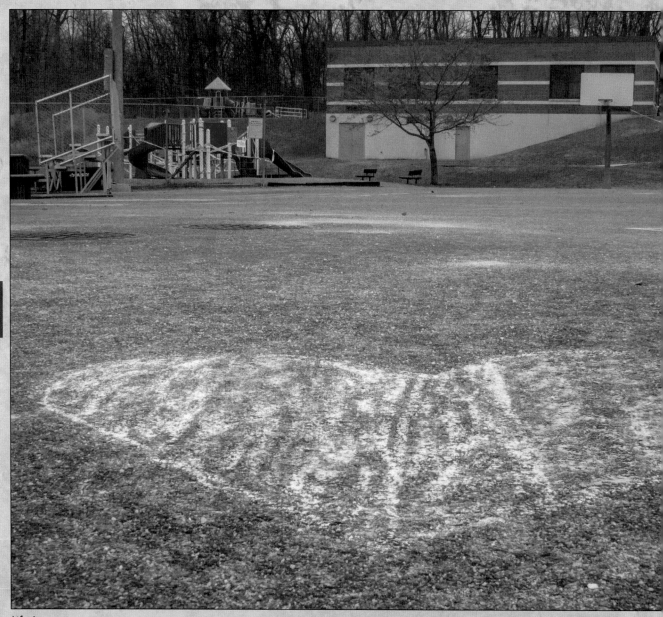

Life Lessons
Closed classrooms, silent playgrounds, and a drizzling rain could not stop little ones from showing
they care at Jefferson School, Summit, New Jersey, March 28, 2020 (Photo by John Ruffley)

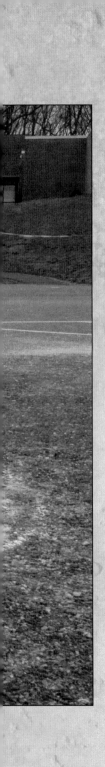

Just Walk

Mary Burns

March–June 2020

At the appointed hour every day, between three and four o'clock in the afternoon, I step out of my house to walk—the one activity that relieves the stress that comes with teaching 106 eighth-graders from my dining room table. While walking, I notice whether the sky is sunny or cloudy. I feel the wind on my face. I soak in my surroundings—trees, birds, chipmunks. I breathe in fresh air and feel my frustrations melt away.

At first we were told we'd be out of our classrooms for two weeks. In that time I received more than three hundred emails from students, teachers, and parents. Most students were doing their work. I was encouraged.

Quickly, those two weeks extended to the end of the school year. I just kept going, beginning work at 8:00 a.m. sharp and continuing until 2:30 p.m. Most days I didn't stop to eat lunch so by the time I quit, I felt nauseous and like my head would explode. Those days, I decided, I'd go for a walk, regardless of the weather. That's how my habit started.

After six weeks it was evident some students were struggling with learning online and managing their time.

The eighth-grade team hadn't even heard from a few students at all. The reasons were varied. A couple were responsible for their younger siblings and expected to teach them while their parents worked. Another student's mother, an essential worker, simply didn't have the time to ensure her sons did their schoolwork.

We teachers asked the school resource officer to check on some students at their homes. We found out that one had told his mother the school year was over. Since English wasn't her primary language, she'd been unable to understand the information the school sent her. The resource officer quickly remedied the situation.

With only three weeks left in the school year, I tried teaching some basic genetics. I spent hours finding a video to help the students learn the terminology and do a Punnett square. To review the information, I scheduled two Google Meets for each class; fourteen of 106 students showed up. I scheduled two more drop-in sessions for anyone who wanted extra help; nine students took advantage of my offer.

My frustration rising, I went for a walk.

Some students performed in stellar fashion, though. One, who'd been failing before online schooling, had risen to the occasion. I called to tell her I was proud of her. She thrived in the quiet of her house without the distractions of a classroom. Another student, diagnosed with COVID-19, started feeling better and made up all her missed assignments.

With two weeks of school left, I got so stir-crazy that I decided to meet a friend and walk the rail trail instead of my neighborhood streets. It's an easy walk and I enjoyed being enveloped by the forest. We walked about five miles. On the way back to the car, my right foot began to hurt. I stopped, took off my shoe, and shook it, thinking a small pebble was causing the discomfort. I continued to walk but felt no relief.

It was still painful when I got home, so I took off my shoes and socks and inspected my foot more closely. There was a blister on the bottom of my foot. Surprised, I inspected my sneakers and saw the bottom treads were very worn. *Like my nerves*, I thought. Worry set in. *How will I continue to walk away my stress without a good pair of sneakers?*

I can't even buy a new pair. The store where I buy my sneakers is closed. It's deemed nonessential. I don't agree. My walks help keep me sane during this unprecedented time. I deem my sneakers essential to me.

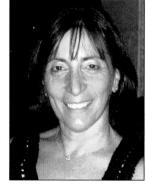

Mary Burns, a mother of three and a teacher, is the author of *Saving Eric: A Mother's Journey through Her Son's Addiction*. She has been involved in addiction advocacy since her son's death. In 2017 the New Jersey chapter of the National Council on Alcoholism and Drug Dependence honored her as an advocacy leader.

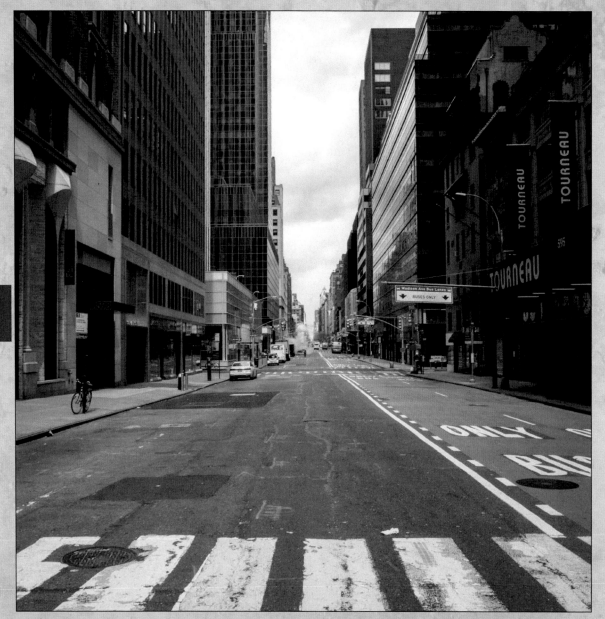

Desolation
Madison Avenue and Fifty-Seventh Street looking north, Manhattan, April 10, 2020 (Photo by Walter Wlodarczyk)

COVID-19 and the
Already Socially Distanced Inner City

Marguerite Dunne

While the Centers for Disease Control collected data, the Upper East Side escaped to the Hamptons, and Mayor de Blasio rehearsed his photo ops, Harvard, whose endowment is $40.9 billion, sent students home in early March. It also accepted $9 million under the Coronavirus Aid, Relief, and Economic Security Act. Later, after being excoriated by the federal government, the university declined the funds.

So went the headlines in the early days of the COVID-19 lockdown. Yet the press hardly mentioned my inner city students who'd given their all to get into Union County Community College (UCCC) in New Jersey, the gateway to the rest of their lives. Everybody at our school doesn't have a bright red school sweatshirt. Some even have trouble affording the books they need for class.

While most Harvard students returned home to their bedrooms with an Internet connection and parents still planning summer vacations, nearly half of UCCC students didn't have computers at home. To them, "just go home" did not have the same meaning. Even though they may come from the low-rent education of public schools, they're still eager and bright and want to play by the (evasive) rules of enfranchised American culture. They ask questions such as, "What does it take to be middle-class-ready?"

Our enrollees are mostly inner-city students of color. Some have learning challenges; some are young single mothers.

Some are adult learners who had stepped away from completing their educations earlier because they needed jobs to help at home.

Some dodge bullets on the way home or walk two miles to sleep in a shelter because a raging alcoholic "stepfather" just beat them up and the only thing they have to hang onto is getting their degree.

Some students go home to a family with a mother, father, invalid grandma, an uncle and his third wife with three stepchildren, another unemployed auntie, and an older brother who liked running the streets during the COVID-19 lockdown because it was such fun facing down the law.

Where was the quiet corner for the UCCC budding scholar to work in? They'd made it to college with the requisite academic paraphernalia when the anomaly of the COVID-19 pandemic lockdown of 2020 suddenly drained their momentum. Having grown up in the inner city, I know the diligence it takes to see a project through is not a value frequently demonstrated on unswept ghetto streets choked with garbage and in building hallways stinking of urine. It takes ingenuity and staying power to navigate the disruptions of homelife and these neighborhoods when transitioning into a serene academic setting.

At our college there are classrooms of computers and lecture halls with overhead screens connected to readily available Internet resources. Designated computer laboratories and libraries on all three campuses allow each learner to write and research. A more-than-willing staff of smiling librarians love answering questions.

There's also an academic success center, a tutoring place where students can go and simply announce, "Help." It's open from early morning until late night and on weekends. Advisers, peer tutors, and professors abound, ready to offer support.

In the rumbling 1960s, Ivy League-educated sociologists described my students as "culturally deprived." For many of them, school is their respite, *the* place where someone is telling them, "You can do it. Here are the tools."

But the politicians' orders took this all away. Forty million Americans lost their jobs. Many of my students juggled an overtime work schedule and extra online assignments to make up for lost hours in the classroom, all while enduring family dramas that rival episodes of the Kardashians and *Jersey Shore*.

We Zoomed some classtime and shared stories about fears for the health of a favorite grandparent, the frustrations of rearranging the already fragile work-school balance, and the effects of mounting bills. One student wrote in our chat room: "Cuomo only cares about people who are dying. People are losing their jobs, starving, and getting evicted. People will die regardless if we stay quarantined or not."

Their stories were immediate, painful, incredible testimonies to the spirit of survival. We tried sharing good moments—the little signs posted in neighbors' windows that read "Be safe" and "We are in this together," anecdotes about shopping for an elderly neighbor, stories about a friend who babysat while the student finished typing a term paper on a borrowed laptop.

We will stay connected after COVID-19, and again, my students will rise. They are masters of finding hope.

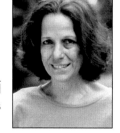

Marguerite Dunne has been a college professor (nutrition, herbology, and English) and a clinical herbalist for more than thirty years. She has had her own radio show, grades papers, and enjoys wildcrafting in the Hudson Valley, New York.

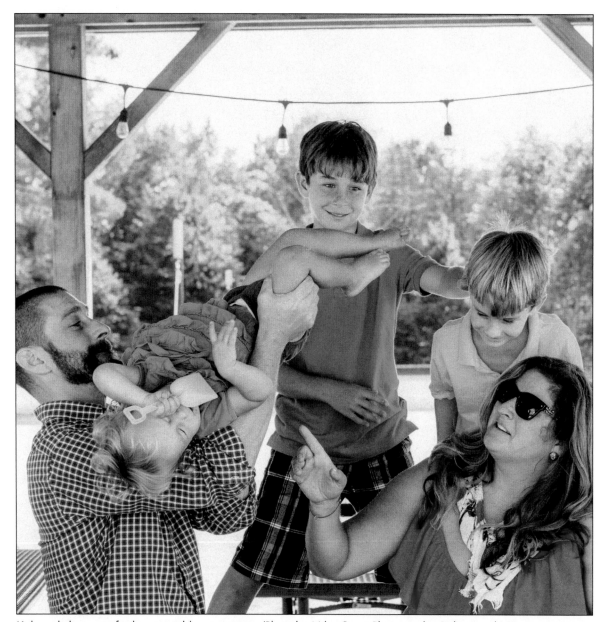

Kids and chaos, perfectly acceptable companions (Photo by Miho Grant Photography, Ridgewood NJ)

Pants Off

Katie Tarta

Whatever was hard before is harder now—work, parenting, marriage, mental health, teaching, addiction, loneliness, death, self-care, forgiveness. All the stressors are magnified and nobody has their pants on.

In my house I'm being watched by a variety of bare-bummed babes, innocently judging, absorbing, sorting into their own perceived realities. Very possibly, I will be the topic of conversation in therapy years later when they can say, "I blame my mother, but there was a pandemic." I hope the latter will vindicate all the errors I've made this season, though in truth they aren't very different than those I made previously, just all the more frequent.

We are a 24-7 family now. No schools, childcare, sitters, sports, camps, playdates, sleepovers. No pants. And no breaks. We are at full throttle here all day (and night) long.

I always appreciated the effort of teachers, especially knowing full well how much goes into helping nontraditional learners. My reading-challenged elementary kid may be one of the few people who, despite an aversion to shirts, has managed to locate and wear one, losing lower torso apparel in the process.

He excels in this pandemic platform where word problems are read aloud, providing freedom to breeze through the math that previously held him back. These gains come at a cost, though. I am now an uncertified special ed aide and have not been nominated for tenure. God bless the teachers, especially those gifted with patience, a category unto itself potentially deserving a purple heart.

School's done, thank God. Sixth grade happened in the dark corner of my basement, perhaps apropos to those who have survived it and maybe easier in retrospect. My middle schooler sat curled in a fleece blanket, wearing only a T-shirt and socks, in my mini home-office space, no longer needed after the Payment Protection Plan installment pay from my employer ran out and my job was eliminated. Previously, keeping this kid off screens was my "mom goal," but he needed screen time to grade up. Managing how to appropriately utilize screens educationally, socially, and for entertainment turns out to be a much more complicated endeavor than just limiting time. Where is the manual? It's exhausting. The pre-COVID days when I failed to engage his interest in non-pixelated activities now look like a three-hour Minecraft binge. But the bar has fallen even lower. Accomplishing any kind of self-care, whose definition has become quite loose, requires a sitter and, frankly, screens are the closest thing to having one. Those three-hour-video-game days pale in comparison to what is now indulged so I can bathe or even just drink a hot cup of coffee alone.

The preschooler who looks at Disney+ sees hours of villains and princesses, stories that outline a fantasy world whose boundaries to reality were faded. Knights in armor saved Aurora, Rapunzel, Snow White, Cinderella, and even Ariel. Right up until COVID, a rescuer was coming. Obvious now, even to a three-year-old, is the reality that Dr. Fauci is no knight and he will not save her from our new isolation.

Traditionally scolded for poor representation of society, Disney has incorporated more shades of the human race and challenged the rescue figure. Unlike my generation, who grew up waiting for Prince Charming, my daughter is fully aware that guy is not going to save her. Deluded she won't be. She is, however, doused by a bit of heartbreaking reality. We seek hope together wearing Moana and Elsa costumes, without any pants, as we sing along and wonder just how far we will go, after all.

Here's the secret, 24-7 families are pantless—not the business-on-top, party-on-the-bottom, Gen Z chic-kinda pantless. The 24-7 family is pantless in a frazzled, out-of-time, out-of-laundry, scraping-for-creative-ideas and prioritizing-needs kind of way. Often these needs are determined hourly. We're living the addicts' version of parental survival, one moment at a time. School's out and jobs are different; some are working more than ever, some not at all. In my house we have both and a whole host of new problems.

The hope for the future isn't a neatly laid out plan by the government or even the modified ten-year track we role-played in premarital counseling some decades ago. The problem is, the plan was shredded, set on fire, and given a cyanide pill. So, where is the hope? It's in our willingness to pivot again and again and again. It is trusting that we are not alone, that there is a God and a purpose. It is the Divine story, the American story, the parent's story: we adapt, we change, and we do it falling forward.

Summer 2020: may it be the respite families need for act two because if nothing else, we learned it's not going back to the way it was before. No more Prince Charmings. No more underappreciated special ed teachers. No one-size-fits-all pediatrician recommendation for screen time. This is an all-hands-on-deck, activating-all-thrusters, new kind of busy. We aren't overscheduled anymore, but free calendars are full with parenting, with or without pants.

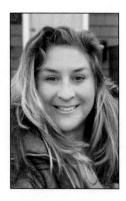

Katie Tarta, BS, MBA, is a corporate planner, realtor, recruiter, and lifelong learner. She is a storytelling, Christ-following mother of three partnered to her best friend for twenty years and still treading. Forever grateful and humble, she refuses to refute or be held hostage by a host of life hurdles. She and her family live in Bergen County, New Jersey.

QUARANTINE

Dealing with COVID-19 meant living in isolation and, occasionally, if we'd been exposed to the virus, under self-imposed quarantine. Our homes were sanctuaries but also fortresses as we watched our neighbors come and go. Those of us in suburbia passed our neighbors while walking, often crossing a street to avoid breathing on each other. Those of us in city apartments took extra care in public spaces.

VOICES
FROM AN
EPICENTER
Page 141

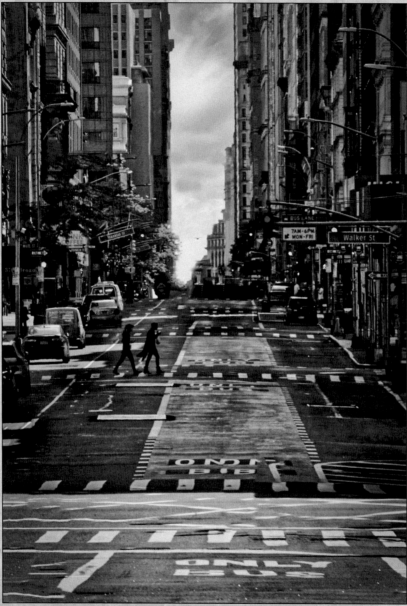

Treading Through Tribeca
Two pedestrians cross a desolate street in Tribeca on Memorial Day during the
lockdown, May 25, 2020 (Photo by Ellen Bedrosian)

Constant Zigzags

Lisa Coll Nicolaou

March 2020
On my street
we have two nurses
and a physician's assistant
who heads the ER in Hackensack.
One lives to my right,
one just across the street and
the third to the left
of our little white house
at the end of a small
cul-de-sac in a place
called Radburn, in a town
called Fair Lawn, in the
densely populated
state of New Jersey.
When those English architects
designed Radburn, a planned community
with winding paths and large shared
parks and small plots of land,
did they realize that one hundred years
later the residents would be able to stand
at their little front porches and safely
wave to each other as they clapped

for their healthcare workers at a safe
social distance?
Each morning, the first thing I do
is look out my window to see whose
car is gone.
If it is Emma, at Hackensack hospital,
then all day long I think about her,
wait to see her Jeep, which she drives too
quickly, something that used to bother me
in our life before, until she returns home
to her baby daughter.
If it is Maya, who leaves at 6:00 a.m.
for her twelve-hour shift at a hospital
in New York, I stand at my kitchen
window at dusk and stare silently until
she returns to our street.
John is on a different rotation
and because he is my age and the most at risk,
some days I do not have the courage
to look to my left to see if his car is missing.
My other neighbor is a chef.
Once we were Girl Scouts together,
her mother our troop leader.
Chris is a good scout and deserves
every badge as she shops for the nurses,
and cooks for the elderly.
She leaves treats at my door,

a can of roasted nuts for my husband,
fresh fruit for me, ice cream for my daughters
and most mornings, I leave a pitcher
of iced tea on my porch for her,
place it as an offering before I take
my morning walk, a thread to my survival.
Each day follows the same route but changes
from the constant zigzags to remain six feet apart.
I marvel at the boldness of the chipmunks,
count the cardinals and identify the woodpeckers
whose sounds puncture the silence.
Every day I search for a little miracle.
Today I stopped at the basketball courts,
the hoops removed, and watched a young
ice skater practice her spins on the asphalt.
She spun so effortlessly, almost flying,
and watching, I was momentarily buoyant, too.
A moment of magic in a time of worry,
a lot of gratitude to live in a place with parks
and birds and friends and neighbors.
A whispered prayer to make it through another day.

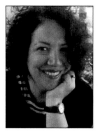

Lisa Coll Nicolaou has lived in Radburn, a historic community in New Jersey, for most of her life.
After many years of inspiring her students to write, she began to write poetry late in her life. In
2016 she won first prize in the Allen Ginsberg Poetry Awards for her poem, "My True Religion is
Kindness."

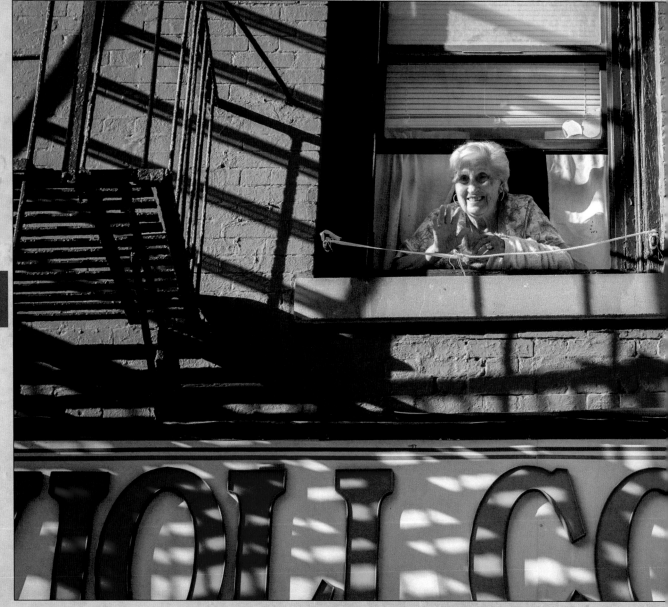

Quarantena
Little Italy, May 3, 2020 (Photo by Walter Wlodarczyk)

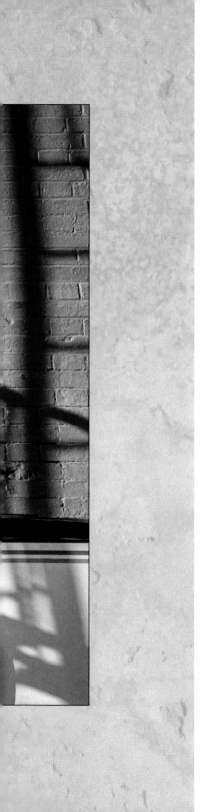

A Conversation at the Railings

Michael Luongo

May 3, 2020

I am behind my neighbor as she moves up the stairs. Every breath is a fight, which is normal for her. She has far too many health conditions and isn't much older than I am, ticking a little past the half-century mark. When she turns to look at me, I notice her mask is more complex—white, thick, covering more of her face—than the one she wore the last time we were on the staircase together.

A few steps in her wake on the worn marble staircase, I am cautious as I draw breath through my own blue surgical mask. I know I could easily pass her, as she sometimes tells me to do, if these were normal times. For the now, I am okay being a little behind her.

It's the railing I am looking at, too, with caution. She has used it every step of the way to pull up her frail body as she fights gravity to ultimately make her way to the fifth floor.

Her mother is the same age as mine, eighty-eight, and our conversation centers on ensuring they are protected. Unlike my mother, hers isn't tucked away in suburbia. Rather, she's here in Washington Heights, perhaps one of the most deadly places in all the world to live now.

"She hadn't been out in weeks," my neighbor says of her mother, "but she went down this morning at 6 to feed the cats." They're all cat ladies, the ones who live above me. "It was the only time she could walk down the stairs and know that there would be no other people around."

The conversation then centers on the clinic where my neighbor goes, part of what we still call Columbia Presbyterian, as does everyone in New York, though it's no longer the hospital's official name. She says she was told that more than half the families who are clients have someone infected with coronavirus.

"There's whole families, eight of them, all packed into a few rooms in already too-tiny apartments. One gets it, and then they all get it," she says.

We live in an immigrant neighborhood, still, even with massive gentrification and displacement. We're both sure that whatever numbers are being reported, they have to be higher. We know even in her own family, a relative was sick one day, dead the next. There was never a visit to the doctor, never a way to know what she actually died from. But all the symptoms were there.

That leads us to talk of the geriatric center a few blocks away where nearly one hundred seniors had died of the coronavirus—one out of seven residents. My neighbor also tells me that various others from our building had lived out the last part of their lives at that geriatric center. They'd died long before the pandemic but what she said made me realize how close a connection we all have. These long hard-worked immigrants who'd fled a revolution on their home island had finally moved when this 1890s walk-up was too much for their ancient bodies. My neighbor, her sister, and her mother are the last remaining residents of one of those families who lived in the building when I first came here some twenty-plus years ago. Back then several apartments belonged to different branches of the same extended family that had escaped Castro's Cuba.

We soon arrive at my own landing. As I open the door, we continue to talk, and then her sister bounds down half a flight, giving a joyful maskless hello.

We then talk about our mothers' birthdays to see which one technically is older than the other, even though their ages match for now. I tell her to tell her mother hello, knowing it's not safe anymore for me to do it in person.

I walk into my apartment's long hall, throw down the bags of groceries, one with overpriced bleach, strip my clothing, scrub my hands. Soon after, I call my own mother.

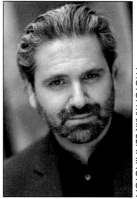

PHOTO: MARK BENNINGTON

Michael Luongo is a freelance journalist and photographer living in New York and an online writing instructor for UCLA who has taught previously at universities in the United States and China. He has authored or edited sixteen books, primarily on travel, including *The Voyeur*, a novel loosely based on his time as an HIV researcher in the 1990s. He was a 2016 University of Michigan Knight-Wallace Journalism Fellow. In July, 2020, he joined New York City Health + Hospitals COVID-19 Test & Trace Team as a Community Engagement Specialist. Twitter @michaelluongo; www.michaelluongo.com

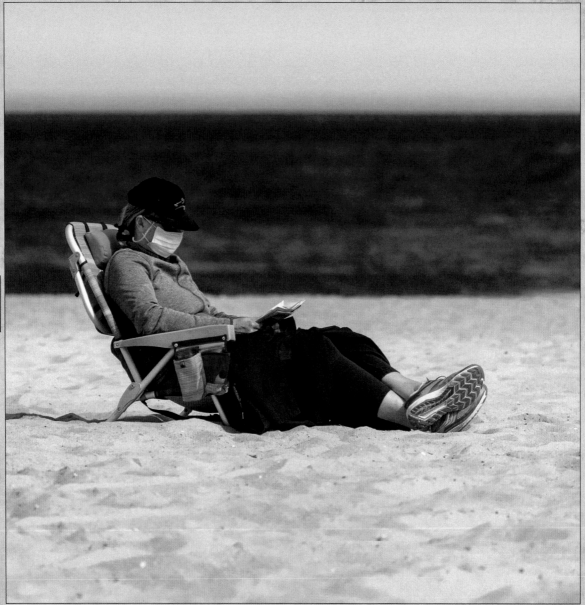

Making the Best of It
A lone woman takes in the fresh air as New Jersey beaches re-open, May 7, 2020
(Photo by Jessica Margo)

Diving Six Feet Deep

Victoria J. Perry

June 16, 2020

I

Being house-sheltered due to COVID-19 connects my feelings to 9/11. Life as I knew it is gone. I give myself permission to lie on the couch, mindlessly watching television and yet present to my grief. No judgment, or self-chastising for tasks undone, I sit with my feelings of loss and sadness. This virus cancelled the long-awaited trip to Argentina. My clothes for dancing the tango in Buenos Aires, laid out in March, still rest on the guest bed. There is no deadline for packing away the daily reminder that life can change on a dime.

II

I face the fear of getting the virus at age sixty-six. From what I read, due to lack of medical supplies and equipment, if there's one life-saving respirator and two patients who need it—me and a person in their forties—I'll be left to die. I firmly resolve not to get the virus. That solves the dilemma.

III

Some days I feel like it's Christmas morning—excited about what gifts the day will bring! Being in the moment, without any attachment to the next second, is a centering experience. Peaceful. And then there are those times when utterly deep feelings of isolation bring me, weeping, to my knees. I'm no stranger to living alone and I appreciate my own company. Yet I'm finding the absence of physically touching another human being to be the most challenging aspect of the pandemic.

I feel grateful to walk outside, six feet apart, with a friend at least twice a week. For six miles of walking or hiking we exchange ideas. I interact with the energy of another person. We're both so careful about not touching that when I step over a fallen tree, he reflexively reaches out to support me and I pull my hand away, nearly tumbling in the process. I'm deeply concerned: will I ever be able to touch someone without fear of getting the coronavirus?

IV

The beaches at the Jersey Shore are open though the boardwalks are closed to the public. My daughter, Trisha, invites me to sit on the beach with her family, keeping our distance. I jump at the chance to see my grandchildren whom I haven't seen in six weeks. My heart feels energized watching them do cartwheels in the sand while I talk to my son-in-law about what's going on at his job. Lucy, their goldendoodle, snuggles up to me. Taking a risk, I stroke her light, honey-colored coat. Pure ecstasy. Much too soon my granddaughter, Grace, is hungry and they're leaving to go home. No eateries are open; all nonessential public places are closed. When we get to our cars, I'm not prepared for my deep sadness. I can't hug them. Runaway tears roll down my cheeks.

Cody, my nine-year-old grandson, says, "Grandma, I want to hug you and I know I can't. So because my mother came from your belly, I'm going to hug *her* and that will be like hugging *you!*"

Cody and my daughter wrap their arms around each other. Witnessing their embrace, I feel heartened. Cody playfully continues, "Besides, you both smell good!"

We wave our goodbyes. Sliding into the driver's seat, an inner dam bursts and I release six feet or more of uncontrollable sobbing into my car.

V

I have a profound realization about grief: when someone dies, the way we grieve has to do with an unanswered question. Maybe all grief contains unanswered questions.

After my husband, Dennis, died, my question for him was, "Did you love me?" It propelled me to travel uncharted inner and outer territories. Receiving the answer, I knew in the deepest part of me that our story was put to rest.

VI

In these days of isolation,
my heart expands.
Self-awareness and compassion flourish.
Blessings, insights, and presence
deepen.
Relationships with another
are my opportunity to grow and reveal the path to self-love.
Resting in the heart of the Divine,
I surrender to what is.
A prayer to myself emerges,
and deeply I ask for forgiveness.

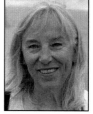

Victoria J. Perry worked as a psychotherapist. She lives in Long Branch, New Jersey. Prior to the pandemic, her time was spent with family and friends, dancing, traveling, writing, and painting watercolors. Her current writing project is a book of micro-memoirs.

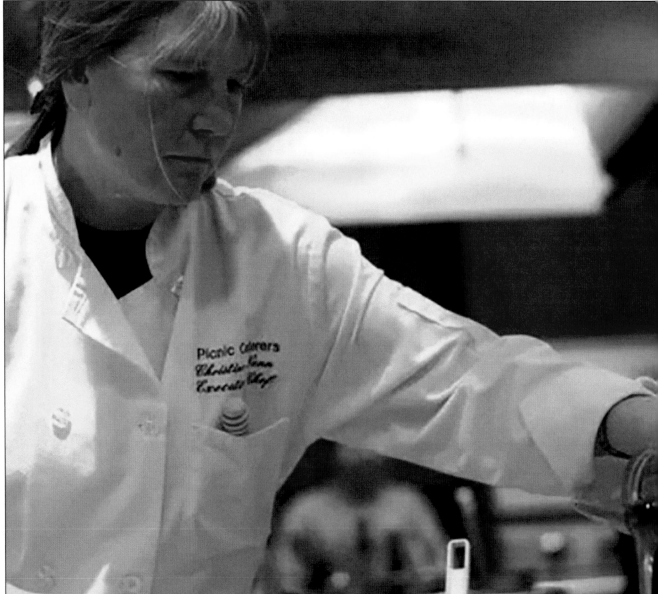

Chef Christine E. Nunn participating in a culinary competition (Photo by Jason Perlow)

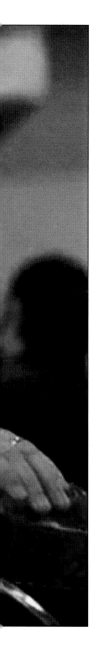

Old Wisdom in a New World

Christine Nunn

April 6, 2020

Hi Mommy,

As you are certainly aware, I'm living in a crazy world down here. I've been thinking about you a lot lately. I've decided to deal with the current world pandemic the way I assume you would. You were part of "The Greatest Generation" surviving the Great Depression, World War II, and the loss of so many. You entertained yourself with a good game of bridge, a good book, and a good cup of tea.

Me? I'm trying to read, but for the first time in a very long time, I cannot concentrate on my book—and it is a good one. Tea? All day, but, boy, at 5:00 that changes to wine. Bridge? The closest I've come to a game that uses your brain is taking mindless quizzes on social media as I scroll aimlessly and time passes.

But, trust me, I am trying. You always said, "Money can't buy you happiness" and darned if you weren't right. Listen, when I had money it bought me lots of happiness. I traveled to amazing countries and cities and dined out (my favorite hobby) at some of the world's greatest restaurants. I went to bars with good friends and quaffed way too much Veuve Clicquot. Guess what? If I had all the money I wanted, I couldn't do those things now, so you were right in the end. Money cannot buy you happiness.

You know what it can buy? A lot of groceries. *A lot* of groceries. Listen, you also said, "Pick yourself up, dust yourself off, and start all over again." Have you seen how my industry, the restaurant business, has tanked and will, I guess, continue to tank for upwards of a year? Well, you were right again. Instead of being chef for a new restaurant that was supposed to open last month, I am cooking for vulnerable seniors who are on oxygen or suffering with heart failure or other ailments. I deliver them low-sodium and other dietary-restricted meals that otherwise would be difficult for them to get. Does it mean I have to go out to the store? Sure. But heck, better me than them, right? So I'm making a modest living and feeling darn good about it.

How about, "What's done is done"? I keep trying to figure out when the sanitizing is done. I come inside, take a shower, throw my clothes in the laundry, and then decide I am dirty again because I touched my clothes. So I wash up again, touch a bottle of wine, wash my hands, sanitize the bottle of wine, and then wash my hands because I touched the bottle of sanitizer. Oh, it is never done, Mom.

And what about, "Tomorrow is another day"? Now, more than ever, it sure is another day I am beyond thankful to be alive and healthy. It is also another day of the same old same old, for the most part, though I did start to teach myself the drums and I can flute a mushroom like nobody's business. And yes, my clients are eating plenty of mushrooms—very sexy-looking mushrooms.

And, I am embarrassed that you were wrong when you said, "No one can ever take away good manners." Oh, Mom, yesterday, while wearing a pair of twenty-year-old pajamas and standing next to a dishwasher full of dishes, I chugged milk out of a gallon bottle like I was an animal. But, worry not, I still cross my legs at my ankles and say "please" and "thank you." I won't mention those fried bologna sandwiches on white bread I've been eating.

You taught me to go out to the garden to relax. "Get a little dirt under your nails," you said. Listen, Mom, every nice day I head out to the garden, but dirt under my nails? I am washing my hands every ten minutes on the 1s, like the traffic report for 1010 WINS. But you'd be pleased to know that right next to the daffodils you planted, chipmunks have built a nest. And I have the time every single day to check on them and wish them a happy day. Oh, and indeed the garden centers are open for business and I hope this is the year my garden is half as beautiful as yours always was.

"Treasure the simple gifts," you would remind me. I got a great gift recently— two bottles of hand sanitizer. I treasure them. But, most importantly, I treasure a gift you gave me—the reminder that "patience is a virtue." That's for darn sure.

Love, Bug

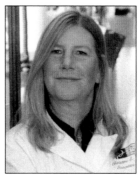

Christine E. Nunn is an award-winning chef and food writer. She is the author of *The Preppy Cookbook* (HMH, 2013).

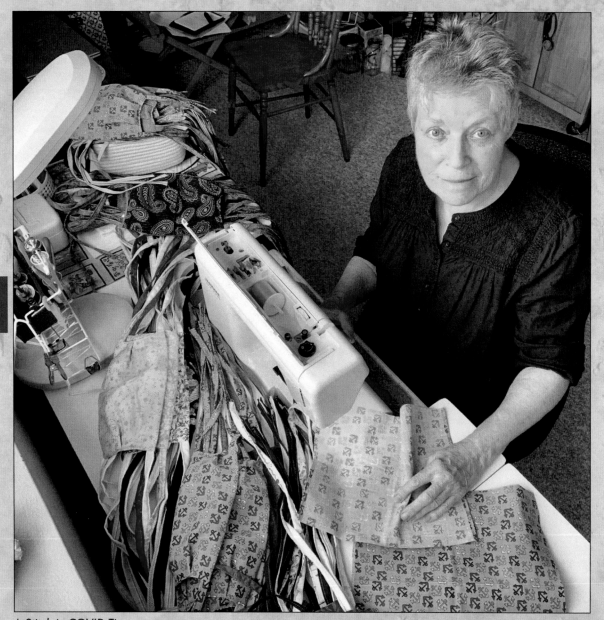

A Stitch in COVID Time
In Rockaway Township, New Jersey, MaryEllen Renard has switched from dressmaking to face mask production in response to requests from area hospitals and nursing homes in desperate need of Personal Protective Equipment, March 25, 2020 (Photo courtesy of MaryEllen Renard)

RELIEF

COVID-19 taught us to find new, simple comforts in a world where our usual pleasures and cultural events were no longer available. We learned new ways of nurturing relationships, stayed in closer touch with nature's rhythms and beauty, tended our gardens, and became culinary adventurers in our kitchens. Dinner became a nightly celebration. We also relished the companionship of our pets.

VOICES
FROM AN
EPICENTER
Page 159

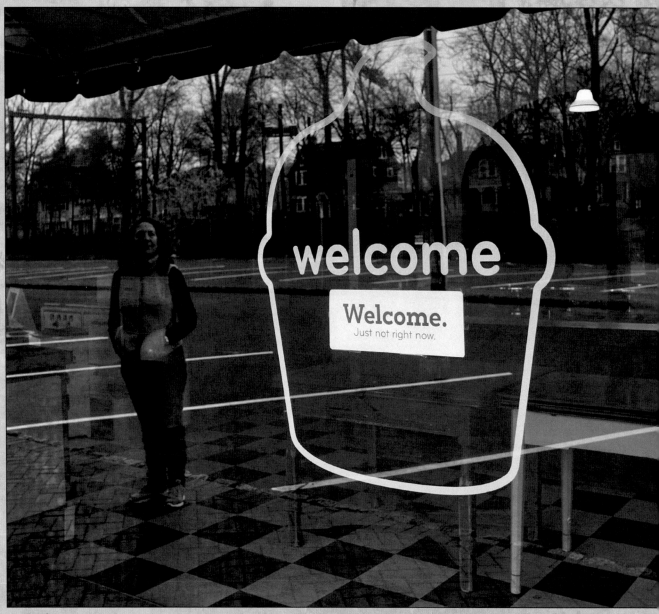

Not Right Now
In the first couple weeks of the state shutdown, Joyce Andrasz of Maplewood comes across one of
the town's closed shops, The Able Baker, March 29, 2020 (Photo by Tom Andrasz)

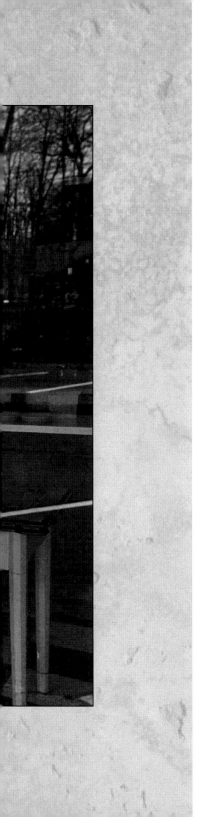

Succor for Sorrow

Elizabeth Berin

June 28, 2020

My husband and I, like most people we know, live in voluntary isolation. Our children are grown and live far from us. Our friends are quarantined in their own homes and may as well live far from us. We stay at home except to shop for essentials such as food, gas, and stamps or to stretch our legs on our street or on a sparsely populated section of rail trail. Our other outside activities are suspended.

We work at our professions only if the task is something we can do from home. We have no commutes to the office and no meetings in a conference room. We do no big box shopping and occupy no seats at performing arts events, ball games, or even at the table with family and friends for holiday celebrations. Absent these usual activities, we fill a lot of time with Netflix, Zoom meetings, housecleaning, and cooking.

The fact my husband and I are over sixty lands us in the category of "COVID-vulnerable." We take all the precautions we can to stay well. They've worked so far. I know we're lucky but we could still contract the virus sooner or later. Each new day has therefore become important and I try to give it content, to make it distinctive for us and distinguishable from those that preceded it.

When I wake up each morning, my first thought is how I'll make the new day meaningful. Seen through that lens, televisions, computers, and housecleaning seem mundane. But food is another matter. Food brings a measure of joy. It stimulates our deprived senses. We can see, touch, smell, and taste our meals.

In quarantine, we've elevated our meals. Why save the good china? Use it. Got table linens, candles? Use them. And why not eat foods we'd sworn off pre-pandemic when we thought we'd live longer if we ate "right"? These days we gnaw on charbroiled red meat, savor fish chowders made with heavy cream, fork-wind pasta covered with a red sauce that has simmered on the stove for many hours, spoon mashed potatoes made with cream and butter onto our plates, slather baguettes with mayonnaise dips, and drink wine to wash it all down.

And we save room for desserts. Nothing is too rich for our palates in quarantine. It sounds hedonistic but, frankly, planning and executing my meals is a highlight of every day. It's a solitary activity made for a solitary life deprived of other small pleasures.

Food is also love. Six weeks ago our son had his forty-first birthday. I was hard-pressed to come up with a gift or a way to celebrate him. He lives twelve hundred miles from us. I don't know what he wants that he doesn't already buy for himself. Even in normal times, any gifts we give him seem to disappear into the ether of his life. But he does miss my cooking. So we hit on the idea of preparing a virtual birthday party for him.

We set the table with our best porcelain, candles, flowers, a linen tablecloth and napkins, and an empty chair for the absent honoree. We prepared dishes he likes—steak tartare, roasted beets with burrata and a sprinkling of pistachios, broccolini, grilled bronzini, rib-eye steak, with red wine. We dressed in our finery—a jacket and tie for my husband, a silk shirt and string of pearls for me. We toasted our son with wine in stemmed glasses. We held nothing back.

We even recorded the entire presentation on a video and sent it to him as a gift. The party was for him. No. It was for us, too.

Food and its preparation distract me from thoughts about the family we cannot touch, the friends we cannot see, the opera and theater we cannot attend, the group sports we cannot play. We miss the sight, smell, and sounds of our children, the salt of their kisses. We can no longer hug them or our friends or rub shoulders with people who sit next to us in the public arenas we used to frequent. Family, friends, and strangers are now threats to our lives. Food is succor for our sorrow.

Elizabeth Berin is a Minnesota expat by way of Manhattan. She currently lives in the mid-Hudson Valley. She is a design historian, designer, and writer.

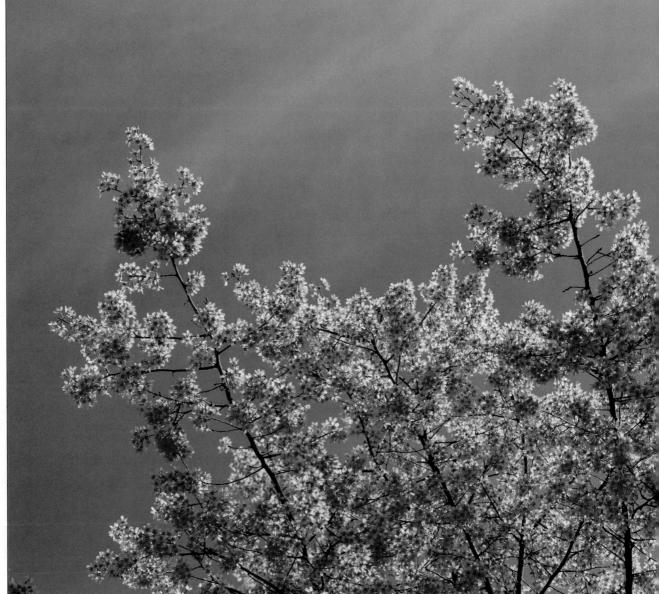

Bright pink blossoms from a Japanese cherry tree bloom against a bright blue sky in Maplewood, New Jersey, during the state's COVID-19 lockdown, March 21, 2020 (Photo by Joy Yagid)

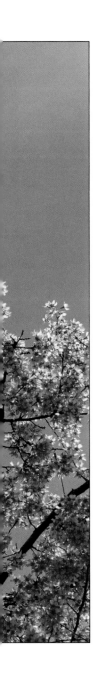

Oh, the Earth!

Maggie L. Harrer

June 25, 2020

It's been three months and five days since I've left my New Jersey home. The play I was to direct in New York City was postponed as was all other work for the foreseeable future.

My husband, a trumpet player, also had all of his work indefinitely postponed. We agree that by the end of 2021, work might be possible. Maybe 2022.

At first the quarantine was peaceful, even freeing. He practiced trumpet as many hours a day as he was able—a longtime wish of his. I spent hours finishing a script I'd been working on for a year—a longtime wish of mine.

Then the headaches started. I was compulsively watching the news about COVID-19 in our county, an early epicenter. The numbers of cases, hospitalizations, and deaths were horrendously large.

Over time, as I watched the news, tension seized my head and neck and my jaw locked. Later, I awakened at 3 a.m. and stared at the ceiling, wondering when the future would be hopeful, or even predictable, again. Always a seven- to eight-hour-a-night sleeper, I got four or five hours, maybe.

I agonized not just about COVID-19 but the complete disintegration of our federal government's response, followed by political outrages, the murders of Black Americans, and protest marches. Then began the violence from our own police, who looked like an invading, militarized force often running roughshod over protesters.

To calm myself I tried exercising, reading, more writing, even yoga breathing. Finally, I decided to just avoid the news. I went from reading three hard copy newspapers and three digital newspapers daily to none.

With vulnerable lungs from childhood asthma and years of pneumonia, I felt it too risky to venture out, even to join the protesters who had my heart. COVID-19 had locked me in.

So I paced my yard which, like Gaul, is divided into three parts. I paced across the front yard, measuring the sun. I marched around the back, evaluating the shade garden projects I'd never completed and the few struggling hostas and lilies of the valley that had managed to reseed themselves.

I peered in the overgrown flower beds. Summer productions always took me away at the crucial nourishing/flourishing time. As I directed far away, my loving, ever-helpful husband mowed my gardens before I returned home. Wanting to get rid of the towering weeds that had claimed them, he accidentally mowed down my plants in the process. Now there were only weeds.

My psyche crumbling and in desperation, I donned full mask and gloves and reconnoitered a nearby garden outlet. The parking lot was empty. I spied only employees. I filled a wheelbarrow with impatiens; a mini rose bush; marigolds, to keep the deer away; spinach and purple eggplants, for my sunny front; basil, Italian oregano, orange thyme, and sage for the border; hostas in rampant purple, rich red, and luscious green; and a sole whimsical fuchsia for my shadowed side garden.

Carefully pulling out my credit card, I swiped it and returned it to a baggie to be sanitized later. Oh, the times we're in. Then I loaded my trunk.

Gleefully, I returned home and arrayed my plants in their new formations. You have to prepare plants by placing them for a few days before digging them in. I hauled out my bright purple hose, bought one summer when I was convinced I'd finally grow my gardens, and watered each one of my recruits.

Then, like a conquering general, I reviewed the troops, adjusted their alignment, and assured them I'd be here all summer to care for them.

Several days later, with hoe and trowel, I plunged my hands deep into the soil. Oh, the earth! That pungent aroma of deep, redolent richness filled my soul. I dug holes just wide enough for the roots, then backfilled and pressed so that each plant was held gently in the earth's embrace. Again and again. At day's end, I peacefully positioned rocks I'd dug up, designing a border between the path and my plants. I bivouacked in my new garden; no encampment could be sweeter.

That night, I slept for eight hours. Oh, the earth!

Maggie L. Harrer is an award-winning director/choreographer, producer, writer, wife to trumpeter Rick Henly, mother to opera singer/film director Katherine Henly, and a passionate storyteller. During quarantine she has completed a coming-of-age screenplay, *Light in Water*, and is finalizing a memoir about growing up as a tomboy in Iowa.

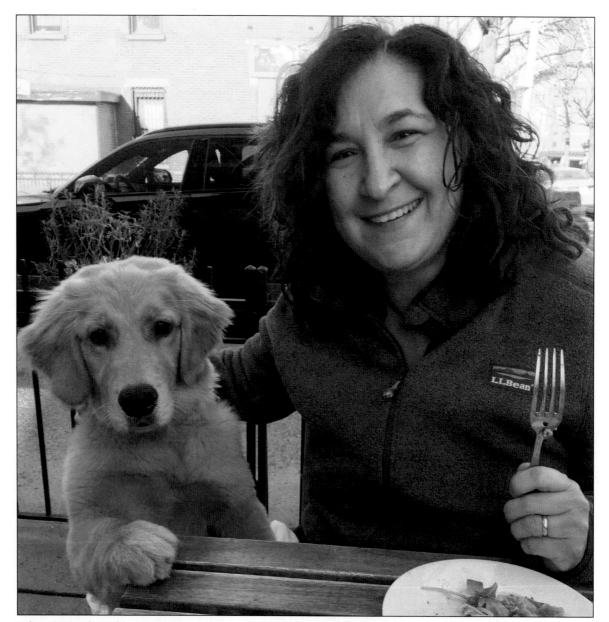

Helene Stapinski and her puppy "Scout" at a sidewalk cafe in Brooklyn in mid March 2020
(Photo by Lisa Bauso)

Scout and Me

Helene Stapinski

Last April when Blue died, I said I needed at least a year to mourn. Blue, our Australian shepherd, was a real character. With his sad eyes and disheveled white wisps of hair coming off his ears, he looked remarkably like Albert Einstein. He wasn't the smartest dog in the neighborhood, but he was the sweetest. And I missed him terribly.

When summer 2019 came around, though, I realized we could up and go wherever we wanted without worrying about what to do with Blue. We flew to Southern Italy, to my family's ancestral town and had a worry-free two-week vacation.

By September, my teenage kids were making a hard press for a new dog. But I wasn't ready to commit. I missed Blue still and loved my newfound freedom. I resisted. They persisted.

"Okay," I said, "we'll get a grown rescue."

"But let's just look at some puppies," they said.

Anyone who has just looked at some puppies knows how that ends. There they were, a litter of ten golden retrievers, all about the size of a loaf of bread, crawling onto our laps.

Right after Christmas, we brought Scout home from her Long Island breeder. Her father was a champion, so she was a true beauty with deep red hair, giant paws, and a wide smile. She also had brains. Scout house-trained in two days. I was embarrassed to tell other dog owners I met, particularly the older couple a few neighborhoods over who had Scout's sister. We had playdates so Banksy and Scout could run and wear each other out.

For a few weeks Scout slept in a crate by our bed. She whimpered and made me curse my decision to get a puppy. It reminded me of the days my son had colic, when I turned my head and everything went by in a weird blur.

Scout ate several shoes, socks, part of the Holy Family under the tree, and a series of earplugs, which swelled to three times their natural size before she expelled them. She ate a bar of soap and threw up all her dog food in a sudsy pile, then took a nap under the couch.

And she kept growing. Fifteen pounds turned to twenty, then to forty-five. Now fifty-five. And I wondered, how did this beast come to live in my house?

And then the coronavirus came to Brooklyn.

Food shopping became a death-defying act. Never-ending sirens left us anxious and worried for who was on the other side of those ambulance calls. Banksy's family moved upstate. Several people we knew died.

And suddenly, there was Scout, strong and beautiful, sleeping through the night and ready and able to handle the horror each day. A redheaded clown with delicate red lashes, she hugged us each morning when we rose from our *Groundhog Day* slumber as if she were meeting us for the first time. And so the new day, which we were unwilling to meet, became new and beautiful for us, too.

When I secretly cry, Scout is there to put her giant head in my lap and lick my wounds.

When my husband needs a break from his constant Zoom meetings, he takes Scout for a spin around the block.

When my kids are frightened and ask questions we have no answers for, Scout inevitably takes their mind off things and makes them laugh. She rolls around on the rug like the puppy she still is. Or steals a face mask and makes us chase her before she eats it whole. She tries to hide under the couch though she can't fit anymore.

Without Scout, I don't know what life would be like in quarantine. There would be so much more tension, fighting, and mourning the life we may never get back.

The days of unfettered travel are long behind us, and likely gone for good. But there are long walks in Prospect Park, thanks to Scout. Just last week, off leash, she pranced and danced around a solitary woman on a walk through a meadow. Because the woman was wearing a face mask, it was hard to tell how she felt about Scout being so close, her paws all muddy, her smile wide but dripping with saliva. As I passed her and tried to get Scout to heel, I felt the woman's smile behind the mask.

"You," she said to Scout, "just made my day."

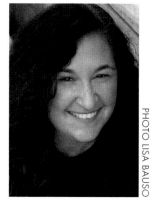

PHOTO LISA BAUSO

Helene Stapinski is a journalist and author whose latest book is *Murder in Matera: A True Story of Passion, Family and Forgiveness in Southern Italy.* She lives in Windsor Terrace, Brooklyn. www.helenestapinski.com.

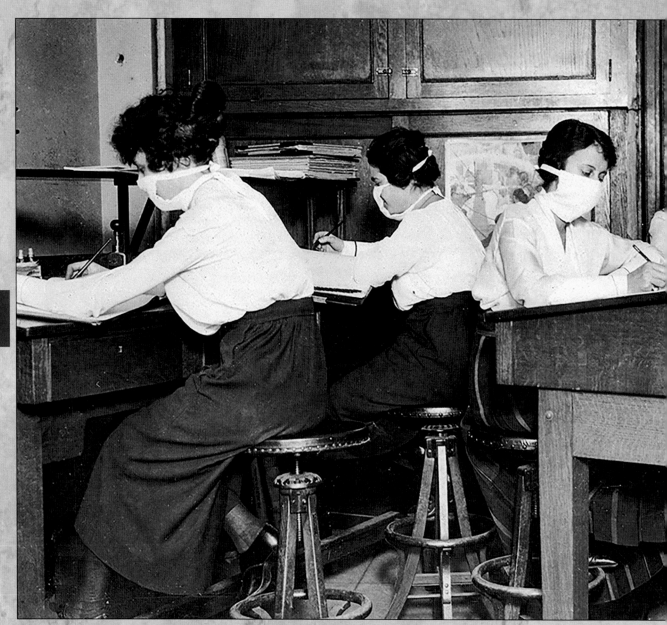

CORONA
CITY
Page 172

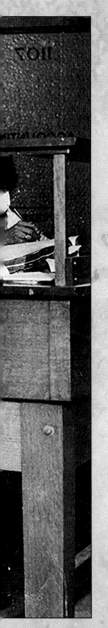

HISTORY LESSONS

Looking for direction and facing an unknown future, we turned to the past. Humanity had endured other plagues. Books and articles about the Bubonic Plague abounded. So did discussions of the 1918 influenza pandemic, which killed 675,000 Americans. Many of us posted pictures of ancestors who'd died in that pandemic. For others, dire times brought back memories of post-World War II Europe. We searched the past for survival tips and inspiration.

VOICES FROM AN EPICENTER Page 173

Everything Old Is New Again
Photograph 165-WW-269B-24; "Medical Department – Influenza Epidemic 1918 – Masks for protection against influenza. Girl clerks in New York at work with masks carefully tied about their faces," October 1918, American Unofficial Collection of World War I Photographs, 1917–1918; Records of the War Department General and Special Staffs, Record Group 165; National Archives at College Park, College Park, MD.

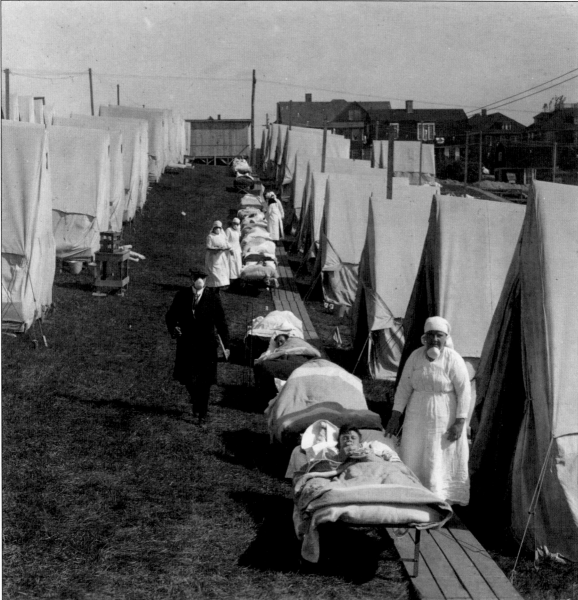

Photograph 165-WW-269B-19; "Medical Department – Influenza Epidemic 1918 – Emergency hospital, Brookline, Massachusetts, to care for influenza cases," October 1918, American Unofficial Collection of World War I Photographs, 1917–1918; Records of the War Department General and Special Staffs, Record Group 165; National Archives at College Park, College Park, MD.

Promise of Sunlight

Kristina Lloyd

April 20, 2020

Due to several long-term illnesses, I am high risk for COVID-19, which sparked intense anxiety. It's not that I fear death. What terrifies me is the idea my husband and children wouldn't have me here to love them every day.

Then I saw a picture of an open-air hospital taken in 1918 during the Spanish flu pandemic. In the photograph patients take in sunlight as they lie on cots alongside several white tents in a field. Back then medics found that patients nursed outdoors recovered better than those treated inside. *Is this true?* I asked myself. I discovered it is. Science has proven those medics right: sunlight is germicidal and fresh air is a natural disinfectant.

These two simple facts made me feel better. They gave me hope.

For five months I'd been hiking at a local state park in Sussex County, New Jersey. My health greatly improved, as did my mobility and attitude. Every day I looked forward to entering the forest and winding my way toward amazing views of New Wawayanda Lake. Depending on the weather, the lake has a hundred different appearances. In fog it is misty white. In rain it has so much texture. When raindrops hit the surface, they make small moving circles. Snow and ice carve a smooth thick layer over the top that looks like a mirror for the clouds.

The forest is another treat. Halfway in, there's an ancient pine grove where I always take a deep breath and inhale the aroma. It clears my lungs and urges me onward.

On challenging weather days the park is mostly empty. When it's sunny and warm, there are a lot more visitors. The parking lot overflows. Pet owners let their dogs run free when they should be leashed. Trash is left behind. People do as they please.

After COVID-19 was announced, visitors were told to social distance. Early in the morning and on cold, rainy, cloudy days, we everyday visitors respected this mandate. We honored the landscape and kept safe spaces between us. When we saw someone walking toward us, we stepped off the trail and kindly let them pass.

But the crowds poked fun at the new rules. They congregated in groups. Teenagers lay on blankets together in the fields. They kissed and hugged and rolled next to each other as if there were no risk at all. They seemed to mock the virus with their healthy young bodies. They scared me. I gave them a wide berth as I walked past, unnecessarily holding my breath.

Because of the mandate to shelter in place, more people were staying local. It was still allowable to walk in the park with proper social distancing—keeping six feet apart. But more folks flocked outdoors. The parking lot was not the only thing overflowing. So were the trails and roads. There was no room to maneuver around the crowds. One day I decided not to get out of my car and risk exposure to the virus.

Forced to stay home, a feeling of melancholy enveloped me and did not evaporate. I wasn't the only one who noticed the rule-breaking masses. The governor closed the state parks. Most national parks had already been closed.

As days and weeks go by now, I miss my hikes in the forest. My body creaks without daily exercise. My lungs crave fresh air and deep breaths. My walking shoes, left in a corner, wait for my return. The streets around my house are too narrow to safely traverse. The woods behind the house are too steep and craggy. I try driving to a town park that hasn't been closed yet but it's just not the same. I can't hike six miles into and out of the woods, up and down the mountains, and around the lake. I even miss the cold rainy days, the muddy trails, and the wayward dogs. *Will my lungs expand again to meet the day? Will I survive this?*

I force myself outside to walk up the hill to get the mail. As the sun pokes through the clouds, I think of the teenagers on the blanket in the field. Do they intuitively know the powers of the sun are healing? Is this what pulls them together without caution? I want to feel like that again. I want to be free spirited, healthy, and loved without fear.

I wish I could return to my carefree self and just enjoy the company of friends. That's what I really miss. I'm afraid I'll never feel like that again.

I decide to drag a cot onto our deck with a pillow and a blanket. I lie down and reacquaint myself with the sun, just like those patients in that old photograph. When the quarantine lifts, I will be so ready. The forest beckons. I hear the trees whispering my name.

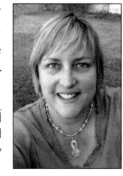

Kristina Lloyd was born and raised in Northern New Jersey, where she has been writing and making art since she was able to pick up a crayon. Her writing has been published online and in local newspapers and magazines. Her artwork is in collections worldwide. She is currently working on her memoir.

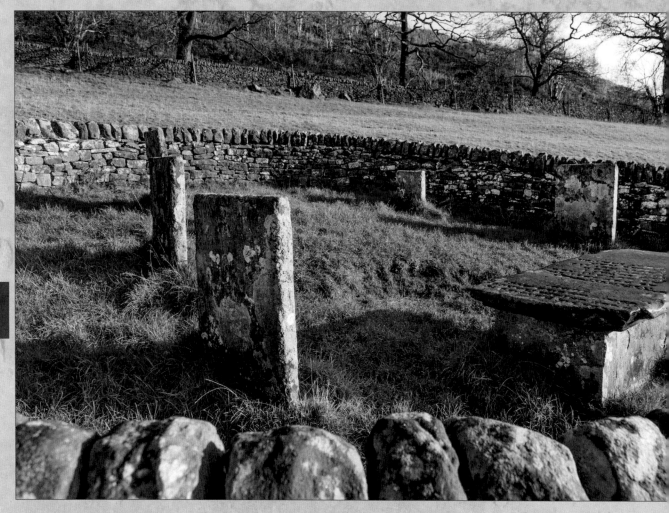

CORONA
CITY
Page 178

Epicenter Again
This small graveyard outside Eyam in Derbyshire, England dates to 1665/66 when bubonic plague ravaged the village. Eyam residents quarantined. For food and medicine, they placed shopping lists on the outskirts of town and left money in "plague stones," which were drilled with coin-sized holes. They filled the holes with vinegar to disinfect the currency. Neighboring villagers shopped and left the items at the site. Social distancing worked. The plague didn't spread beyond Eyam's borders. Lessons learned then are paying off now. COVID-19 has come to Eyam.
(Photo by iStockphoto)

A Modest COVID Proposal
(A Satire in the Spirit of Jonathan Swift)

Richard Devlin

April 2020

This is a modest COVID-era proposal for preventing the parasitic elderly, the unemployed and underemployed, illegal immigrants, the poor, the un-white, the disenfranchised, the sickly, the homeless, and all the whiners and complainers from infringing on the prosperity of this great country of ours. The COVID pandemic is God's way of culling the undesirables from his kingdom. One need only look back to history at the course correction of the Black Plague, resulting from divine retribution for the excesses of blasphemy, heresy or fake news, fornication and abortion. Let's take a look at the facts.

Social distancing may be in. But Social Security has been out of hand for some time now. By some estimates, the trust funds that support this frivolous entitlement will run dry by 2035 and, like gun violence, there is nothing we can do about it. But the pandemic is going to take care of all that without us doing a thing. Most people dying from COVID-19 are old. Many have been clogging our hospitals and nursing homes with their chronic conditions and immunocompromised lifestyles. And in God's divine plan the COVID virus takes the oldest and works its way backwards. In fact, some experts feel young people have a natural immunity to the virus, and that's without drinking bleach.

The future is bright. But let's face it, the old, frail, and unproductive are draining the system by drawing the most from the public dole and not contributing a damn thing. Call it natural selection or just plain bad luck: the COVID-19 virus is taking care of the graying of America and all the burdens to society that come with them.

And the immigrants are on the run. The illegals who haven't been arrested and deported are running for their lives back to their own shithole countries. The rest are dying at home without health insurance. The other foreigners who may have wanted to immigrate to the US of A know now they are safer in their own countries, since we have the highest COVID death rate in the developed world. America is No. 1! The money we save on tracking down bad *hombres* and putting them in internment camps and the expense of separating their sniveling kids can be better directed to building an even bigger and better wall.

It's heartbreaking to see the poor and the homeless in our cities. At least the rural poor are out of sight. But God helps those who help themselves. It's written in the Bible. This is the greatest country on earth and there is no reason why these people can't pick themselves up by their bootstraps. It's just disgusting. But, again, COVID-19 comes to the rescue. It attacks people who don't take care of themselves. They are sick. They have preexisting health conditions. Many are just crazy while others have perpetuated bad genes. Why else would you want to live on the streets? These people are expendable. They are adding absolutely nothing to society. The poor are takers, not givers. For them and their wretched lives, COVID-19 is a blessing in disguise.

Most of the hundred thousand or so people who die because of COVID-19 will be poor, old, or otherwise undesirable. Now what's wrong with that? We can't save everybody.

Look, our country is in trouble. Our elected officials, locked up in their plush quarantine basements, are doing more now to address the nation's problems, which is to say, nothing at all. We have a presidential apprentice who seems more concerned with saving his own ass and arriving at his next tee time. Anyone who attempts to come near him with an idea is tested to make sure they are a Mini-Me and virus-free.

So now it's up to Mother Nature. Our materialistic obsessions have been cauterized by a virus-driven economic shutdown unseen in American history. We are experiencing a Green New Deal without the legislation. Air pollution is down. Driving is out. Air travel is a distant memory. People are out walking and talking, often in nature. Interdependence has been rediscovered and Zooming is a new verb. Home cooking is experiencing a revival. Parents are getting reacquainted with their kids. Friendship has experienced an enlightenment. If any of us survive the president and COVID-19, without the help of medieval bloodletting, we can count ourselves lucky. But then again, we may end up being a nation of preadolescent boys like Piggy, Jack, Sam, Roger, Ralph, Eric, and Simon from William Golding's *Lord of the Flies*, disastrously attempting to govern ourselves.

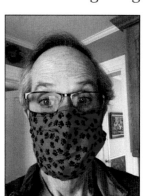

Richard Devlin is a retired septuagenarian living in Red Bank, New Jersey.

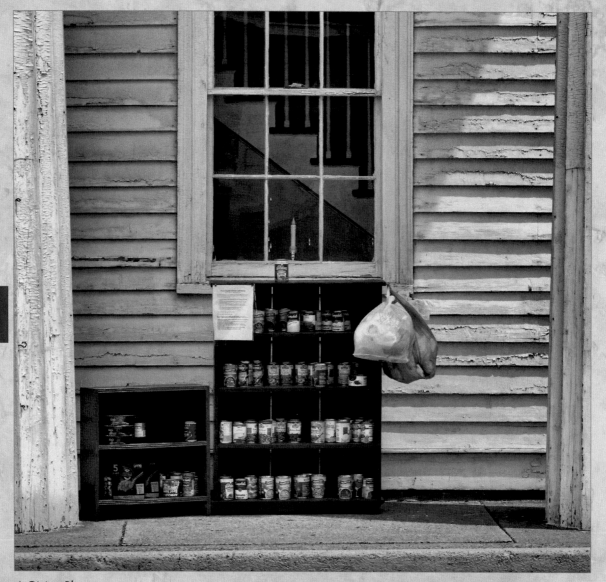

A Giving Place
The Pay It Forward Little Pantry of the First Presbyterian Church in Hackettstown, New Jersey, follows a simple philosophy: take what you need, leave what you can. It is open to everyone twenty-four hours a day, May 19, 2020. (Photo by John Ruffley)

Two Sieges

Robert Reitter

May 8, 2020

Every Hungarian boy is expected to read the thrilling Stars of Eger, a heroic tale, and I was no different. The sixteenth-century story goes like this: A great Turkish force besieged the fort that enclosed the town of Eger, allowing no food to enter. Every day for seven weeks, the force assaulted the fort.

Under the leadership of Captain Dobó, though, the much smaller contingent in the fort held out until the Turks gave up and left. For a boy, the tale was thrilling, in no small part because of Captain Dobó's strong leadership.

These days we are sheltering in place, besieged by a virus that gives no indication of leaving us alone anytime soon. No one knows how long the siege will last or how it will end. And we have no Captain Dobó to inspire us with his strength. It will be up to us, individually, to find the inner strength that will enable our society to endure.

Perhaps that was also true in Hungary in the sixteenth century. Perhaps Captain Dobó is an invention of later writers to capture the imagination of impressionable boys, ready to believe in heroes.

This morning my wife, who does all the shopping for us nowadays, came back from our neighborhood farm store. She reported that shoppers are directed to move in a single line throughout the store now. That way, all masked faces are lined up in the same direction and shopping carts keep everyone a few feet apart. She was taking her time picking up several items at one place, and so holding up all the shoppers winding their way to her. She apologized to those just behind her, but they weren't impatient or angry.

"Don't worry," one of them said. "This is just the way it is nowadays."

Something good may be beginning here, I thought. *People are facing up to their distress and finding calm and strength within themselves they might not even know they had.*

Yet on the two or three days a week I read the morning newspaper, I find so much sad news, it's hard not to weep. So many people, still in the prime of life, are dying. Children are going to bed hungry. Hospital workers are afraid of becoming sick themselves. So many who've lost jobs are anxious about economic survival.

The lockdown only slightly worsens my depression. Far in the past are the days I walked to the train in the morning and walked back in the evening. In between was hard work and a midday break. I'd disappear from my office at lunchtime, have a workout at a nearby gym, and then treat myself to an Indian lunch while reading the book reviews. It's been many years since age and health allowed for all that.

Life without the plague will return as it did after the 1918 Spanish Flu Pandemic and after both world wars. These events have receded into history. One day COVID-19 will be history, too. How will these months of the virus siege look to us then?

I was eight years old when World War II ended and I remember life in the days and weeks that followed. After months of hiding and going hungry, one might think the relief of safety and the enjoyment of feasting would follow. It wasn't like that at all. In those first days after the war I remember the pleasure I took in simple things—a piece of bread handed to me by a generous soldier, a Mass celebrated on a makeshift altar in what had been a bomb shelter only a few days earlier.

Many weeks of hardships followed though they didn't feel too hard to bear after what we'd gone through. There were long treks with my mother on cold March days to reclaim our home in a distant part of Budapest. The very wind seemed to hold something of the fear and uncertainty of wartime days.

Eventually, confidence returned and the memory of fear and hardships faded, though it never entirely passed away.

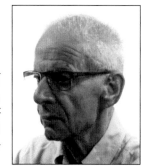

Robert Reitter and his parents immigrated to the US in 1948, having survived the Nazi period in Budapest. Although they'd become Christian, the authorities sought them on the basis of their Jewish ancestry. Once in the US, he attended the Bronx High School of Science and Yale University. He then pursued a career in market research, which he found fulfilling for more than fifty years. In his mid-fifties, he started studying Hebrew and is now a practicing Jew.

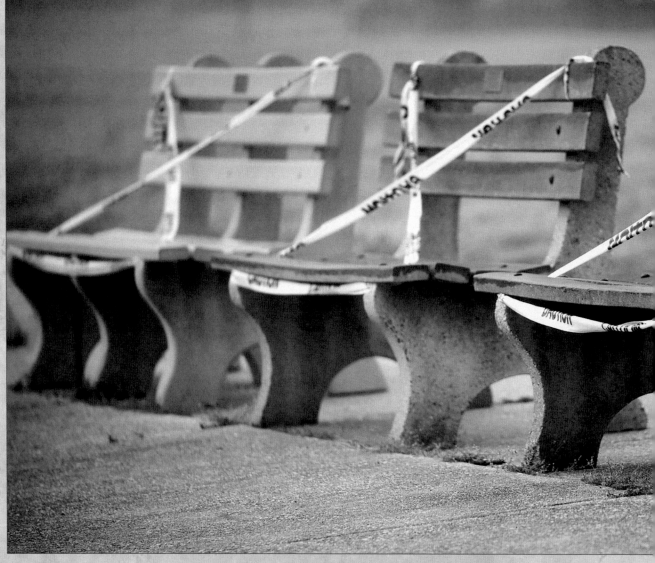

Cautious Beginnings
Benches along Ocean Pathway in Ocean Grove, New Jersey, May 27, 2020 (Photo by Charlene Federowicz)

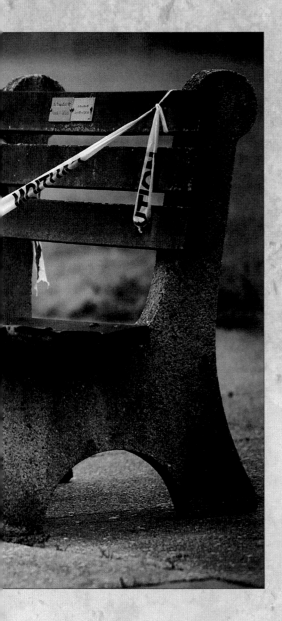

REAL NEWS

Another crisis culminated: we struggled to find reliable, fact-based information about COVID-19. Before the pandemic, corporate business models already had weakened the American press. American newsrooms had lost some twenty-seven thousand journalists since 2008. Parts of the country were "news deserts." Great journalists were still hard at work, though fresh rounds of layoffs and furloughs began. Fake news and politically biased coverage filled the void. So did conspiracy theorists.

VOICES
FROM AN
EPICENTER
Page 187

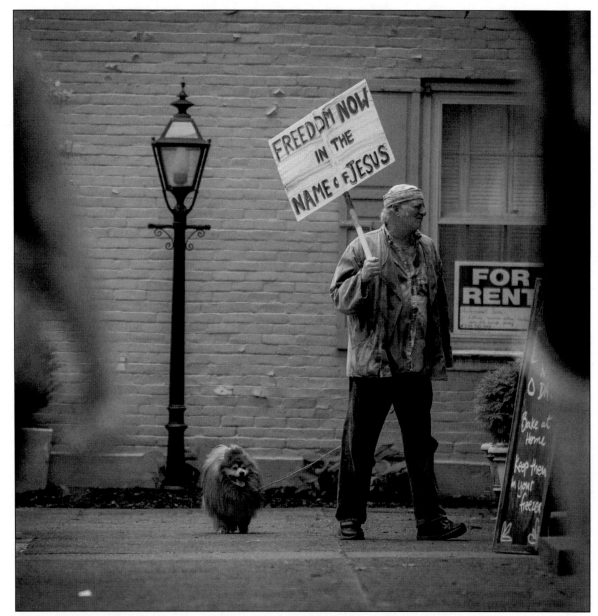

A man holding a protest sign arrives with his dog at an Open Now rally at the Monroe
County Courthouse square and war memorial in Stroudsburg, Pennsylvania, May 15, 2020
(Photo by Daniel Freel)

A Guy with a Camera

Daniel Freel

May 15, 2020

Two-and-a-half months after the *New Jersey Herald* laid me off, I walked down Sarah Street in Stroudsburg, Pennsylania. I was following the sound of chants coming from the town war memorial area: "Open Now! Open Now! Open Now!"

I saw a crowd—a small ocean of red, white, and blue fluttering in the breeze. I stood at the opposite corner, raised my camera to adjust my ISO and aperture, and stepped into the street. The sting of my layoff still showed on my face though it wasn't visible under my face mask. I grew agitated as I looked around and saw no local media present. No cameramen, no reporters or bona fide photographers. *Maybe they're off covering other stories, more important stories. Or maybe there's just no one left in that local newsroom for an editor to send out. Maybe there's no editor.*

A bearded man in his sixties shouted at me.

"Which fake news outlet are you from?" I turned to look at him. "I'm just playing around with you," he said, shooting me a smile.

"I'm nobody," I shouted through my mask. "Just a guy with a camera."

A woman carrying a sign that read "We support small businesses" asked if I was with the *Pocono Record*.

"No, ma'am. I don't think they have photographers anymore." She seemed surprised.

"So, you're one of the people?" she asked, seemingly referring to the gathered demonstrators.

"Not exactly," I said, explaining I'd been a professional photojournalist for more than a decade until the same company that owns the *Pocono Record* recently laid me off. "I'm a citizen now."

"Oh, but you can submit photos to them?"

"I could," I replied, "but I don't think I will."

I understood what freelancing meant: the company I'd worked for would pay me a fraction of what I'm worth and still reap the benefit of my craft. And, of course, I'd get no benefits. I could not agree to that arrangement in good faith.

So why am I here? What's the purpose of photographing this rally if I'm not going to share the images for local distribution? What's the story? What's my story? Do I just want to get out of the house?

According to Pennsylvania Secretary of Health Dr. Rachel Levine, there'd been more than sixty thousand COVID cases in the state and, as of that very morning, 4,342 COVID deaths. Despite these numbers, she reported that over the past fourteen days, there'd been a noticeable decline in the rate of cases. Her report had prompted Governor Tom Wolf to announce that, effective next Friday, a dozen more Pennsylvania counties would move into the "aggressive mitigation" phase of reopening. That phase lifts stay-at-home orders and allows for in-person retail, preferably curbside pickup or delivery.

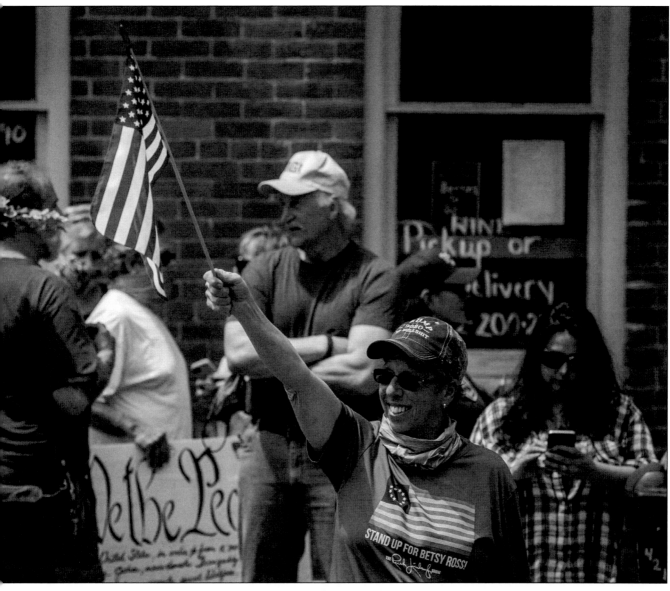

About a hundred frustrated residents gather at the Monroe County Courthouse square to protest Pennsylvania Governor Tom Wolf's stay-at-home orders. Concerned about the local economy, they demonstrate to reopen Stroudsburg's small businesses, which have been closed to in-store shopping for almost two months, May 15, 2020 (Photo by Daniel Freel)

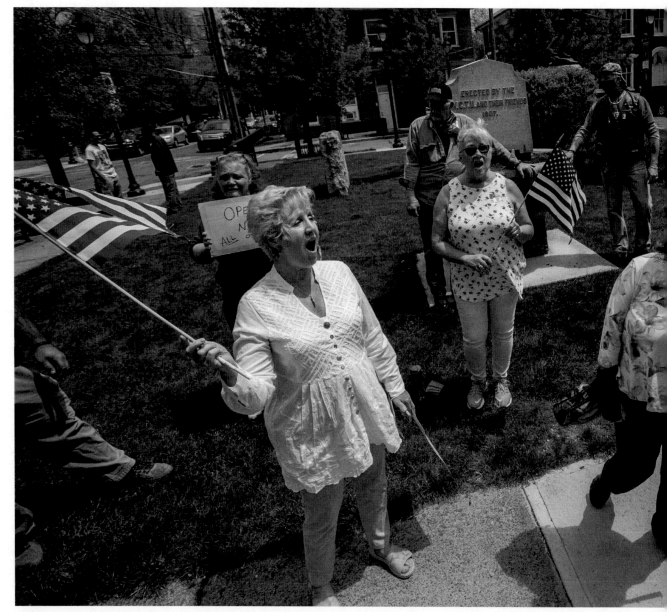

Residents wave American flags and sing "God Bless America" as they oppose
Pennsylvania Governor Tom Wolf's COVID-19 response, May 15, 2020
(Photo by Daniel Freel)

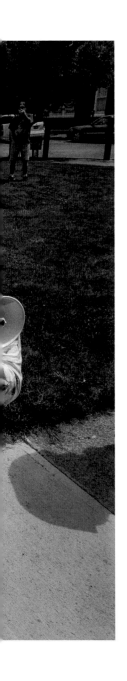

Monroe County, where I live, was in the first wave of counties to be issued a stay-at-home order. I suspected we'd be among the last to lift those restrictions.

So, on a morning when our neighboring counties were beginning to experience breaths of fresh air, a gathering of a hundred Monroe County residents shouted, "Open Now!" The signs they carried condemned the governor.

It was difficult not to confuse the gathering with a Trump rally. There was certainly plenty of MAGA apparel. One man with a long white beard bounced between demonstrators, occasionally screaming "God Bless America" into a megaphone. He wasn't wearing a mask though other Trump supporters were. One wore a mask with "Keep America Great," Trump's 2020 campaign slogan, stitched along her cheek. Other demonstrators seemed to have no political affiliation, though. They carried signs praising Jesus or calling for personal liberty and the opening of the state.

I went to a café window and ordered some chicken empanadas. A voice suddenly called out from behind me.

"There's the only honest journalist left!" It was the bearded man in his sixties again.

"Who, me?" I laughed at him. "I'm not even a journalist anymore. But, you know, I got my camera and I'm just—" I paused. "I'm just chasing the dream."

The words spilled out of my mouth, almost by accident, as I searched for some reason I was there.

Is that what I'm doing now? I used to tell people I was "living the dream." Now I guess I'm just chasing it, whatever that means.

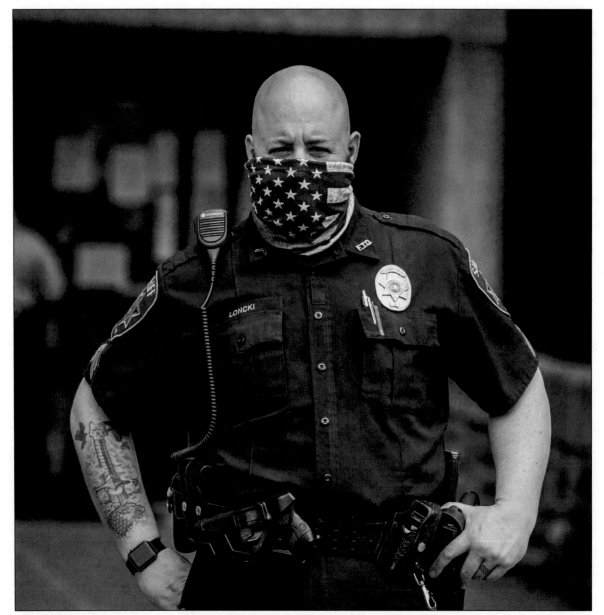

An officer with the Monroe County Sheriff's Department wears a thin blue line American flag bandana as a face mask while he and other sheriff's officers monitor the Open Now rally, May 15, 2020 (Photo by Daniel Freel)

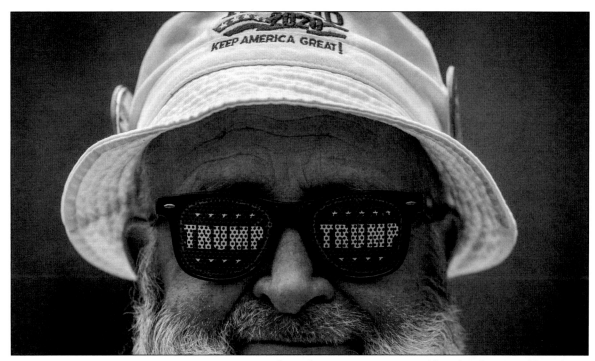

A man dressed in Trump 2020 apparel from head to toe softly smiles at
the camera as he demonstrates, May 15, 2020 (Photo by Daniel Freel)

"Hey man, I'm sixty-five years old," the bearded man said, "and I've been
chasing the dream my whole life. And I'll be chasing it till the
day I die."

I guess that's something to look forward to.

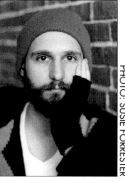

Daniel Freel most recently served as senior photographer at the *New Jersey Herald* from
2011 to 2020, having received numerous awards from the New Jersey Press Association. His
work documenting the pandemic was awarded second place in "Living and Photographing
in the Time of COVID-19," an online juried showcase by The Photographer's Eye collective.
Daniel has a BFA concentrating in fine art photography from Penn State University.
IG danielfreel; Twitter @freelphoto; FB Daniel Freel

PHOTO: SUSIE FORRESTER

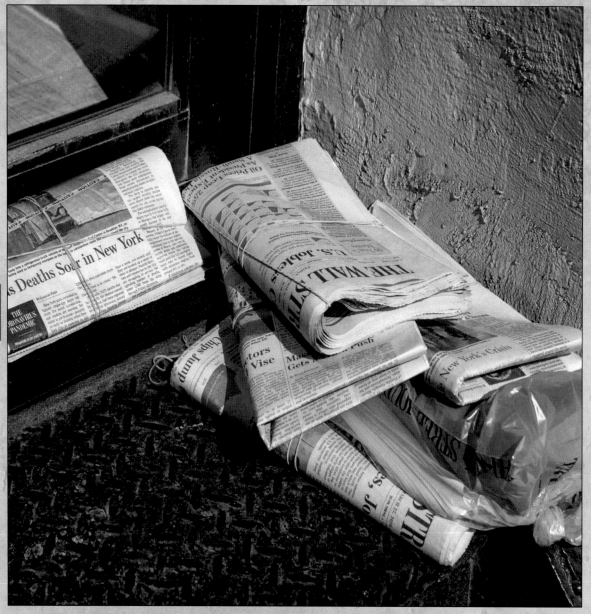

Deaths Soar in New York
SoHo, April 4, 2020 (Photo by Walter Wlodarczyk)

The Death of Informed Opinion

Randy Bergmann

Spring–Summer 2020

I was a victim of COVID-19. Not of the virus itself but of its debilitating effect on the newspaper industry. Ultimately, it cost me my job in May.

After eighteen years as editorial writer, editorial page editor, and columnist with the *Asbury Park Press* in New Jersey—and more than four decades in the business—my number was finally called. Literally. I was told by phone that I was being laid off on my first day back from a weeklong furlough. My first day back was my last day.

I had taken great pride in having survived more than a dozen downsizings during the recessions of the 1980s and 1990s and over the past decade as the steady erosion of advertising dollars whittled away newspaper staffs.

Although the news of my layoff wasn't a major surprise, the suddenness was jarring. And because the staff was working remotely at that point, there were no opportunities for face-to-face farewells. All the goodbyes and well wishes were virtual. There was no gold watch.

Those on our decimated staff—and on decimated newspaper staffs everywhere—were, and continue to be, constantly on alert for signs they might be next. I'd learned eighteen months earlier that editorial page editors and writers working for the parent company were on the short list for the next round of pink slips.

Soon after, I was among those offered a buyout. The terms were unattractive. I passed. As it turned out, I made the right call; that decision gave me eighteen more months to do what I have loved doing my entire career.

Perhaps the most distressing part of being laid off was how it underscored the parent company's apparent lack of regard for opinion leadership. That latest round of layoffs also claimed the only other remaining editorial page editor in the Gannett group's ten New Jersey newspapers.

Statewide today, there are sixteen dailies in New Jersey, fourteen of them controlled by two corporations. There is only one newspaper in all of New Jersey with an editorial page editor.

As recently as the 1980s, there were twenty-six daily newspapers, most of them independently owned. Each had editorial page editors. Each ran at least one editorial daily, offering informed opinions on local issues unavailable anywhere else and holding public officials accountable. At that time New Jersey dailies employed more than fifty editorial and opinion page staffers.

As a longtime journalist who has always believed that opinion leadership was one of the most important roles of a newspaper in a democratic society, those numbers are depressing.

Of course, everyone in the industry has shared the pain of newspaper layoffs. Last year alone 7,800 journalists lost their jobs. The pandemic led to the elimination of another 36,000 media jobs. Between 2008 and 2019, the number of US journalists shrunk by half.

What will I do next? I'm not sure. All I know for certain is that it will involve writing and perhaps public policy and part-time teaching.

Trying to find the silver lining in the COVID-19 pandemic isn't easy, particularly as the virus, once believed to be on its way out, is now surging in the South and West.

Despite losing my job, I feel fortunate. So far, my wife, three teenage kids, and other relatives and friends have avoided the virus. And the restrictions imposed because of the coronavirus gave me the opportunity to spend more time with my family.

For the first time in more than forty years, I went more than two consecutive weeks without working. COVID-19 came when the weather began turning warmer and sunnier and my kids were on an abridged virtual school schedule, followed by summer break. The timing couldn't have been better. I've done more of the things my busy work life had limited—enjoying the outdoors, reading on my back deck, practicing my guitar, and taking long bike rides.

Still, I've experienced daily anxiety about COVID-19 and wondered how far to venture into New Jersey's somewhat reopened world. Multiple times each day, I assess the relative risks that contact with the outside world pose to me and my family.

Effective treatments and a widely available vaccine for COVID-19 can't come soon enough. Eventually, we will get past this. I hope the same can be said for newspapers, print or digital, and informed opinion.

Randy Bergmann was editorial page editor of the *Asbury Park Press* from 2003 to May 2020. Prior to joining the *Press*, he was a national editor for the Associated Press in New York City, editor of the *New Jersey Herald*, and managing editor of the *Princeton Packet*. He has won numerous state and national journalism awards. A native of Westfield, New Jersey, he lives in Jackson, New Jersey with his wife and their seventeen-year-old son and fourteen-year-old twins.

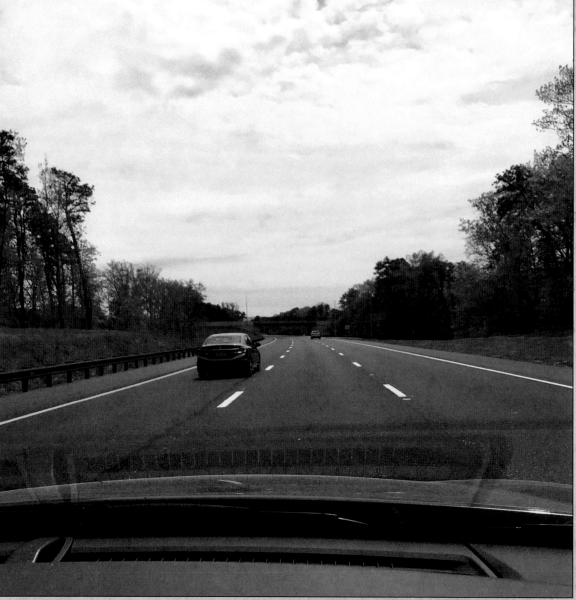

Clear Sailing
A view of the Garden State Parkway headed south toward Exit 44, Pomona, New Jersey, May 17, 2020
(Photo by Donna Grahl)

Journalism by Phone

Scott Yunker

March–June 2020

When New Jersey Governor Phil Murphy declared a state of emergency on March 9, I was six months into my career as a professional journalist. Nine days later, we staffers at the *Coast Star* newspaper in Manasquan got our marching orders: we would all work at home. I poured the contents of my desk into a cobwebbed cardboard box. Another reporter, watching as I lugged my heavy box across the parking lot, said it looked as if I'd been fired. Others took much less. While we shared a sense of relief—the close confines of the office had grown more unnerving each day—I think many, myself included, suspected our time at home would be short lived.

I'd been living with my grandparents, halving the fifty-five-mile commute from my parents' home in Lower Bank, a drowsy, unincorporated village in the Pine Barrens. I decided to stay with my parents for however long the pandemic lasted. Lower Bank, which has no true sense of community in the best of times, would quickly grow to feel even more isolated with the onset of stay-at-home orders.

For me, the first two months of quarantine was a period of stress punctuated by moments of exhilaration. I was the sole journalist regularly cataloging the pandemic in Brielle and Spring Lake Heights. They're two postage-stamp burgs, to be sure, but I felt pride in covering their governments, food drives, and amateur PPE providers.

Those giddy moments of self-importance were drops in a bucket, though. Mostly, I missed the newsroom's friendly racket and I was frustrated that I couldn't be at the scene of any story I covered. Every interaction took place over the phone. Nearly every day I listened to a new voice strained with stress and worry.

Over time grief appeared as residents reported the deaths of friends, long-ago neighbors, and family members. These stories, usually told in confidence, were very few, but they weighed on me. The pain I heard in each voice shook me though people tried to disguise their hurt. We were strangers, after all. Neither of us could put a face to the other's name.

So far, personally, my pandemic life has been marked by privilege and fortuity. I have not lost a loved one to the coronavirus, although I worry for the safety of the elderly in my life. I didn't lose my job. I don't even pay rent. I've experienced bouts of profound loneliness, yes, but the ability to self-quarantine and remain on payroll is a luxury many do not have.

It is now Friday, June 26. One hundred nine days have passed since the governor declared a state of emergency. The past four weeks have been relatively quiet in Brielle and Heights though that could change soon. Summer is here and vacationers and part-time residents may flock to the nearby Jersey Shore, even as withdrawal of federal support closes New Jersey's two federally funded COVID-19 testing sites.

The murder of George Floyd also may spark a reckoning of sorts in these insular, wealthy, and blindingly white communities. On June 13 Heights residents held a Black Lives Matter march. At its July 1 meeting the school board promised, among other things, to emphasize "equity, diversity and inclusion" at Brielle Elementary.

Like many others, I hope the traumatic circumstances wrought by the pandemic can, at the very least, serve as a crucible for dramatic, positive social change. I want to document that change as it occurs and in so doing, further it. The past three months have strengthened my conviction in the constructive power of the written word.

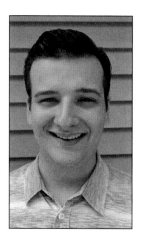

Scott Yunker received the New Jersey Society of Professional Journalists' 2020 Wilson Barto Rookie Journalist of the Year award for his work at the *Coast Star*, a weekly Monmouth County newspaper. He graduated from Ramapo College of New Jersey in 2019.

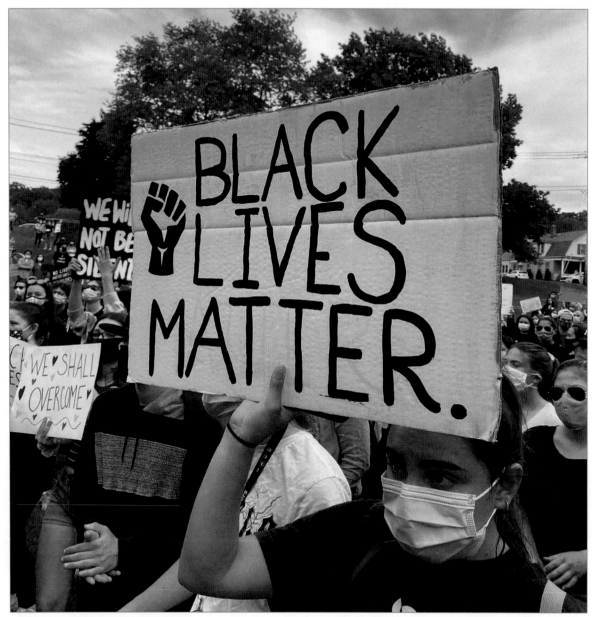

A rallying cry (Photo by Diane Rosano)

Invisible Enemies

Diane Painter Rosano

June 2, 2020

reached for my iPhone on a sunny Tuesday afternoon in early June. *I need to get there. What time is it, for God's sake? 4:07 p.m.? Dammit! It started already. Where's my mask?*

Since COVID-19 hit the Northeast in February, I'd had my college-age son and two younger children at home, all virtual learning, full time. Meanwhile, my immunocompromised husband lived at our summer cottage in Connecticut.

After months of nonstop cooking, cleaning, laundry, grocery shopping, and wiping everything down with Clorox wipes, I was exhausted. That Wednesday, as I sat down to take a break from the domestic grind, my thoughts went to Facebook postings about a local Black Lives Matter (BLM) protest. It was scheduled for that afternoon in Oakland, New Jersey, the next town over. I'd told my kids we would not be attending.

Across the country, protesters incensed by George Floyd's death were gathering in fervor and number. Under COVID-19 quarantine in our suburban cocoon, we watched the news constantly. A steady stream of footage and images from BLM protests gripped us. Rage over Floyd's death and the systemic racism Black Americans have endured couldn't be contained.

But the protests included a faction that descended into looting, destruction, and violence. Earlier that morning women on a local Facebook page had been posting about the Oakland rally:

"I heard they're getting bused in on two or three buses," posted one mom.

"Has the local police department been notified?" another wrote. "I pray there's no looting of businesses!"

"You're not going," I'd told my teens that morning. "I don't want you to get hurt." As I spoke, making the millionth meal under quarantine, news of a Milwaukee protest blared on the kitchen TV.

"I'm not eating in here anymore," my thirteen-year-old said. "I just can't listen to the news." I turned it off, but he still stalked away with a plate of food.

I hadn't worked in a newsroom in years. Yet at 4:08 p.m. the journalist in me activated. I hopped in my car and, donning a mask, drove way too fast up the street. I was headed to the protest. Going felt forbidden. I'd left the house during Governor Murphy's shelter-in-place order, after all. But I had to go.

Amid a stalled economy and unimaginable illness and death across the US, the power and energy behind the BLM movement was mushrooming. My gut told me BLM wasn't a series of isolated protests but rather a powerful wave sweeping the country.

"How can I get to the protest?" I asked a police officer at a blockade near the high school entrance. "I'm with local news." I blurted out the words, completely unplanned. I'd been working on developing a digital magazine for feature stories.

As I opened my car door next to the town green, I heard chants, "Black Lives Matter! Black Lives Matter! Black Lives Matter!" iPhone open, I walked to the center of the action and immediately started filming and taking photos. The leaders were high school kids who took turns standing atop the 9/11 Memorial and shouting through an orange cone to a crowd easily two hundred strong. Social distancing rules were mostly ignored, but I was happy to see everyone wore face masks. The synchronized chants continued: "I can't breathe! I can't breathe! I can't breathe!"

Suddenly, everyone was asked to be silent for eight minutes and forty-six seconds, the length of time the Minneapolis police officer had knelt on Floyd's neck. As I scanned the crowd and saw the eyes of the young protesters above their blue medical masks, my own eyes watered. I felt an overwhelming urge to cry for anyone who'd experienced any injustice or injury because of their skin color.

The dual challenge for every American now is formidable. Brazen acts, such as tearing down statues that symbolize our nation's racist roots, must help us completely excise racism from our society. And we must act together to obliterate COVID-19 from the planet. Unless we defeat racism and plague, two very distinct enemies, none of us will be truly free.

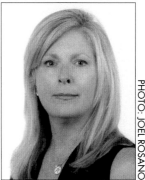

PHOTO: JOEL ROSANO

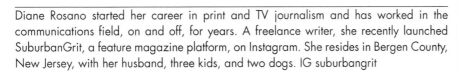

Diane Rosano started her career in print and TV journalism and has worked in the communications field, on and off, for years. A freelance writer, she recently launched SuburbanGrit, a feature magazine platform, on Instagram. She resides in Bergen County, New Jersey, with her husband, three kids, and two dogs. IG suburbangrit

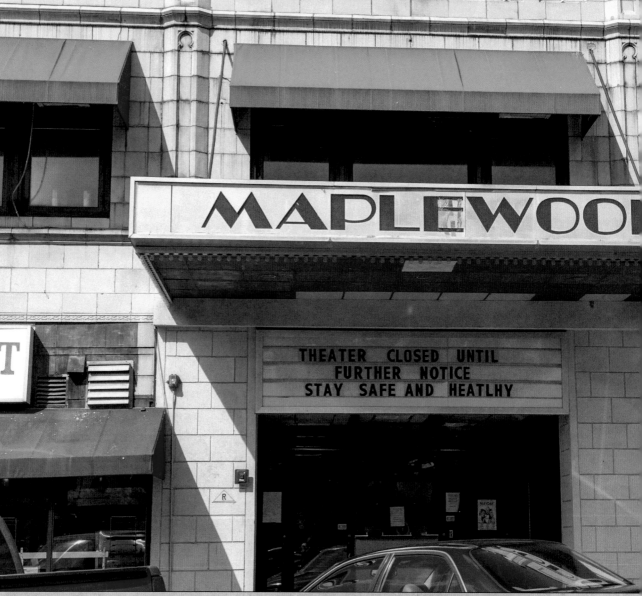

Maplewood Theater
The marquee of the Maplewood Theater, closed due to the state's
COVID-19 lockdown, March 16, 2020 (Photo by Joy Yagid)

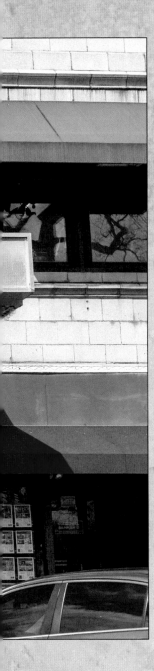

SHUTDOWNS

In the rush to contain the virus, state governments shut down all enterprises deemed nonessential. Those businesses, however, were quite essential to the livelihoods of their owners. Some entrepreneurs had to innovate their way through the pandemic to stay relevant. Others took the time to renovate their spaces. The closing of theaters and artistic venues severely affected our cultural landscape and economy. We mourned these losses, some of which may be permanent.

VOICES FROM AN EPICENTER Page 209

CORONA
CITY
Page 210

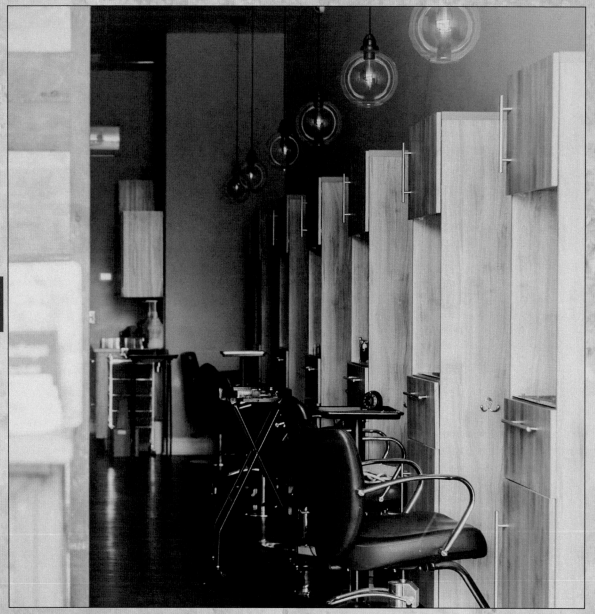

Silent Salon
A once-busy Northvale, New Jersey salon sits empty as a result of the COVID-19 pandemic shutdown mandate.
May 10, 2020 (Photo by Rebecca Osso)

Glamour, Too 2.0

Nic Colannino

March–June 2020

On March 21, 2020 I sat on the stoop of my very modest carriage house. New Jersey Governor Phil Murphy had just announced the closure of nonessential businesses. My stoop is where I go to think whenever the s——t might hit the fan and it seemed like it was about to hit. (NB: "Nonessential" is now right up there with "unprecedented" on a list of words that need to be thrown into the dustbin of overuse.)

What am I going to do? I asked myself. *This is my only form of income.* If I threw in the towel, I'd be giving in—and that means falling into irrelevance. When you own a brick-and-mortar retail shop, irrelevance means death. I am not even programmed to understand giving in! There was NO WAY my Waldwick, New Jersey shop, Glamour, Too, a local beauty product boutique for the glamourati, would become an asterisk to COVID-19.

Pivot. There's another word that deserves a moratorium for at least a year. Everyone was saying, "You have to pivot." Well, if you keep pivoting in one direction, where do you end up? Yup! Right where you started. And I made a pact with myself: when all this was done and we were on the other side, I would not still be sitting here on my stoop in this mindset. I would not remain on hold. Not personally, financially, or spiritually. So I decided to do whatever you call it—waddle, stumble, crawl—forward.

I was going to remain relevant. Forget about making money because I was working three times as hard as I normally do for 30 percent of my normal revenue. But if I could figure out a new way to remain relevant each day, then *that* would be my "new normal." (Toss that phrase into the dustbin, too, please!)

Each day I woke up and asked myself, *How do we reinvent Nic and Glamour, Too?* As my friend Ann so eloquently (cue the eye roll) said, "You will just keep pedaling like a dumb determined ass, like you always do!" She was right. After all, this is the guy who vacationed in Lapland in January.

I love people! So I started by listening to them. More importantly, I heard them. I understood what they needed during this very uncertain time. Early on, with the help of another friend's jocularity and brilliance, we came up with a series of NicKits. I hustled. I created them. I delivered them. I also linked up with a wonderful Instagram personality (shout out to @chezchaya) who was beyond kind to me in publicizing them. Listen, I know NicKits don't change the world. But I also know having gel manicure remover, hair clippers so your man doesn't look like Grizzly Adams, a gentle self-waxing kit, and home hair color kits allows people to feel human even when they have nowhere to go. The kits help my clients feel relevant as well.

And, fortunately, people found me and called to order NicKits. And they told their friends—um, hello new customers—to come to me for their Glamour-ous needs as well. New customers during the COVID crisis. This little shake, rattle, and roll of a pivot at Glamour, Too 2.0 was working.

But ask me what I really gained on the other end of this grueling three-month shutdown and I'd say friendship. Some old friendships were rekindled through this COVID time. I have made so many new friends, too, because those who know my shop know that my customers automatically become my friends.

I know your name and your kids and your friends. I am accountable. I have a face, now with a mask covering half of it. But who cares? On the other side of this crisis, I am still relevant though I'm still not out of the woods ... yet.

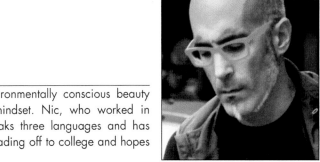

Nic Colannino is a purveyor of ethical and environmentally conscious beauty supplies. His sensibilities stem from his global mindset. Nic, who worked in international governance in his previous life, speaks three languages and has traveled the world. He is the father of twin boys heading off to college and hopes one day to move to the Faroe Islands.

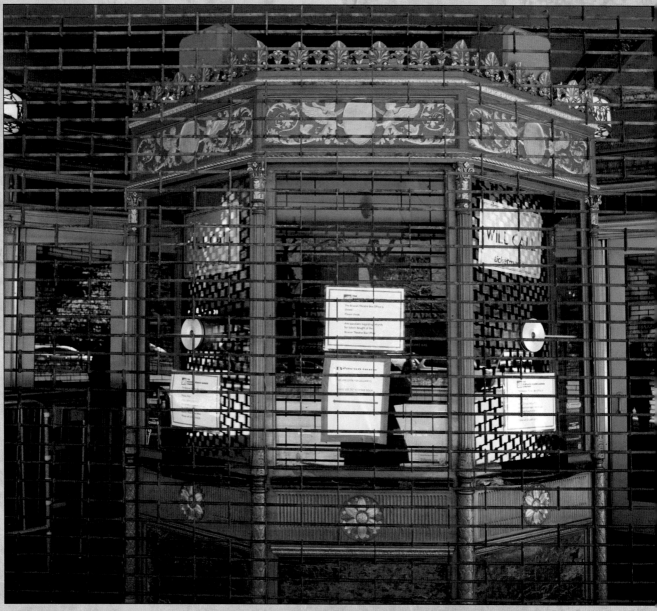

The Beacon Goes Dark
The Beacon Theatre on Broadway in Manhattan is seen
closed on April 14, 2020 (Photo by Christopher Monroe)

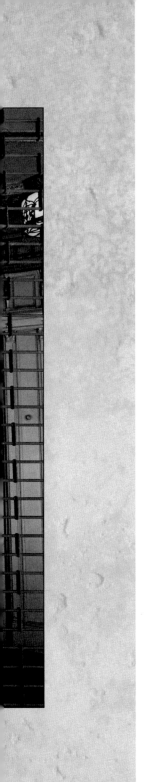

Find Your Light

Katherine Henly

March–July 2020

've called New Jersey and New York home my whole life. My tripod of a family includes my mother, the dancer-turned-director/producer; my father, the classically trained trumpet player who made a career crossing between genres; and me. I never questioned following them into the family business. Music and theater have always made my heart sing.

The hardest part for me has always been the goodbyes—the constant travel, the quick turnarounds for jobs. I continually meet new people with whom I collaborate, build a world and a connection, and open lines of communication, only to break it all down and move on to the next production.

And that's how I came to be in Minnesota in March 2020. The week of March 9 began with a full moon over Minneapolis. I was there to play my dream role of Musetta for *La Bohème* with Theater Latté Da. During the final preview performances, I spent my free time planning my May 30, 2020 wedding to the actual love of my life who, as great luck would have it, was also in Minneapolis. He was in rehearsals, too, playing the lead in the world premiere of *Edward Tulane* with the Minnesota Opera.

We'd gotten engaged in August 2019 after a year and a half of dating across oceans and time zones. There were months apart, layover flights, and lots of goodbyes. Working in the same city for three whole months, right before our wedding, was sweeter than a pool of ice cream.

By Friday, March 13, our world tilted permanently. We both received the news that our productions were shutting down. That night I sang Musetta for the last time to an audience packed with friends and family we'd told to "come now or never." Afterward, I lingered on the dark stage, lit only by the ghost light, to memorize the feeling that remains in a theater—the hum of space once filled with people, connecting.

The first weeks of quarantine, we sang a lot. We danced around our living room, worked a thousand-piece puzzle, prepared music for upcoming jobs, and took on every "challenge" social media sent our way. We even started one of our own—the "La Speranza Challenge," urging singers to hit their best High C. It went viral.

Nights, though, I searched the internet for information about the situation out East, my heart sinking as the coronavirus situation worsened. Bad news came in avalanches: sick friends, deaths, job cancellations, and permanent closures. At first I counted the days. I stopped at seventy-two.

We applied for unemployment and braced for an indefinite future.

We cancelled our wedding; the safety of our loved ones was too valuable to risk.

July 4, 2020

We're still in Minneapolis. Theaters across America are closed. Broadway performances are suspended until January 2021. With no work, friends and colleagues have been forced to leave New York City.

I miss my parents.

I wonder when we'll ever get married.

I wonder what the world will look like for the children we hope to have.

My heart aches for the people, productions, and theaters we won't see on the other side of this. And yet—

One of the first lessons a performer learns is this: find your light. It means wherever you move onstage, or in front of a camera, your job is to find where the light is the most vibrant and beautiful—the most focused. Everything looks better there. Important storytelling moments land better because they can be seen. The simplest gestures become ethereally beautiful and hold a gravity all their own.

To find your light, you must "move until you feel it on your face." That sounds strange. How do you feel something you normally see? I can't answer that scientifically, but I do know that in sunlight or artificial light, there's a little more warmth in the best light. You'll feel it spill across your cheeks, guiding you; and if you close your eyes, the world behind your eyelids fills with a warm glow. It's no longer completely dark.

The light I've found in the past one hundred thirteen days is this: the feeling I love after theater has always been the stillness, the silence that allows the echoes of the music to sound more sweetly and the memory of laughter to resound more clearly.

The world I knew well came to a screeching halt. But perhaps that means there's just enough quiet to hear hope and just enough darkness for that light to stand out. It's our job to find it.

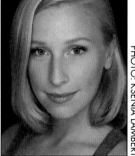

PHOTO: KSENIA LAMBERT

Katherine Henly is a freelance singer, actor, director, and filmmaker currently based in Minneapolis. A short film she directed, *Bones,* premiered at the American Dance Festival's Movies by Movers Film Festival in July 2020. She performed in Operatunity Theatre's *Opera on the 'Virtual' River* in August 2020. www.katherinehenly.com

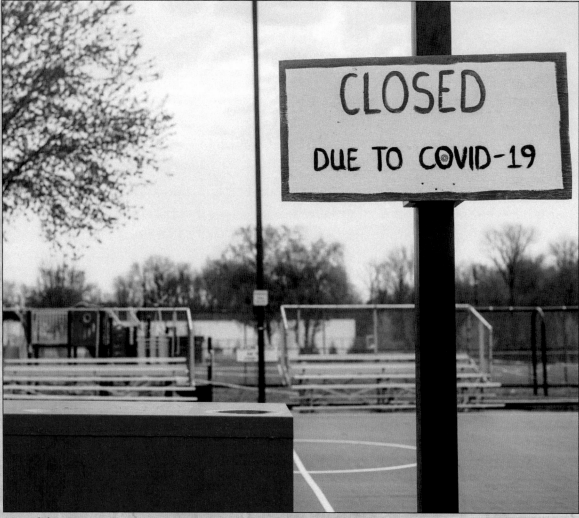

Sign of the Times
Signs and caution tape are posted on a closed Northern New Jersey playground due to COVID-19
shutdown, May 10, 2020 (Photo by Rebecca Osso)

The Great Pause

Linda Mitchell

March 15–May 14, 2020

When COVID-19 cases hit New Jersey in mid-March and the first three cases were announced in Sussex County, I had to let go of the idea that The Tree of Health Center (TTOHC), the natural health and spiritual development center that I co-own, was an essential part of health-care. It wasn't easy. We not only give preventative care but take care of clients who come to us for emotional, mental, physical, and spiritual well-being.

My business partner, Debra, had already decided to work from home. Her work can be done remotely. Since massage, CranioSacral Therapy (CST), and Reiki are my specialties, things were different for me. Massage and CST are hands-on therapies; clients are used to experiencing these services on location. A qualified practitioner can perform Reiki, an energy therapy, remotely, though, and clients are receptive to that.

Forced to be home, I caught up on administrative tasks. Though I don't get paid for doing them, I relished the idea of getting caught up. Tasks can pile up when you're running a business and have an active full-time healing practice. I was grateful that I get Social Security benefits. It covered rent and a few other bills. After that, though, there's not a whole lot left over.

So, diving into this new normal, the first thing I did was apply for unemployment. I hadn't yet filed my 2019 tax return. (That was one of those administrative tasks.) The online directions for unemployment benefits were clear: if you showed your 2018 tax return, you would qualify for unemployment. Relieved, I filled out the online application for benefits. Done. Then I waited for someone to approve my application.

God only knows how long that will take, I thought, realizing that many nonessential businesses were starting to close or had cut back on staff.

On March 26, 2020 I caught a headline in the *Wall Street Journal*: "Record Rise in Unemployment Claims Halts Historic Run of Job Growth." More than three million workers had filed for jobless benefits as the coronavirus hit the economy.

I was one of three million workers applying. Everything on the news was about COVID-19. Knowing I was not in control, I did my best to stop worrying. I waited till the following week to go online and check my claim status. Navigating the site was tricky as it reflected the newest updates and protocols. Finally, I pulled up my claim. Status: unchanged. I was on hold.

I tried calling the unemployment hotline. For a week. To no avail. I decided to give it a break. My health was not worth the frustration.

So many had been affected by the virus in the days leading up to closing our center. That first night I lay in bed thinking, *Is this what depression feels like? Am I depressed?* Knowing I had no place to go, no idea how long the pandemic would last, or how long I'd be out of work, I thought about the world, people I knew, and people I didn't know who were ill, dying, unemployed, or on the front lines. I felt helpless. After all, I was a healthcare provider, a caretaker, someone who always worked every day of her life. Till now.

Waves of sadness, anger, and hopelessness filled me every day. They broke me open. I recognized in myself the stages of grief, learned from my nursing days—denial, anger, bargaining, depression, and acceptance. The world was forever changed. There would be no going back to pre-COVID-19 life. Nor did I want to.

All my life I'd gone through my own traumas and emotional fears about not being enough. This pandemic, finally, was giving me time to be with myself, to pause, to feel, to validate, and to begin my own healing from the past and the present moment of uncertainty.

I didn't hear anyone talking about their emotions, though, and knew I needed to begin the conversation. I started with the TTOHC Reiki Gathering, a group of Reiki practitioners that I needed to move onto Zoom, a virtual platform. A new learning curve for me. At our first virtual meeting I spoke about the waves of emotions that had me questioning if I'd always been depressed. It was great to hear that I was not alone, that others were experiencing their own emotional trials.

It took a pandemic to get all of us to pause. At sixty-seven, I'm grateful to have this time to release some of my old patterns, emotions, and feelings and discover more about myself.

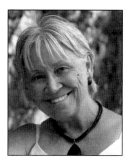

Linda Mitchell is founder, partner, and director of The Tree of Health Center in Newton, New Jersey. She is working on a memoir, *Saving Daisy.* https://www.ttohc.com

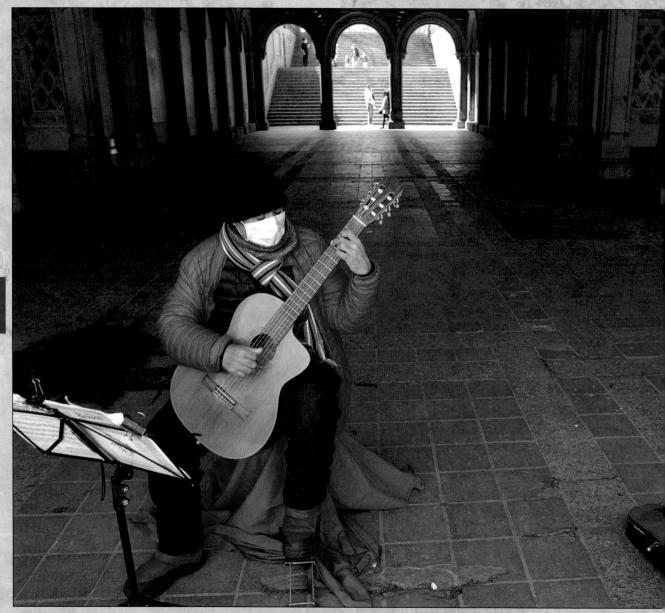

Better Angel
A busker plays in the empty Angel Tunnel in Central Park on April 25, 2020
(Photo by Christopher Monroe)

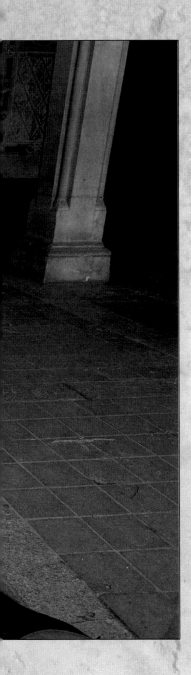

STATES OF MIND

The pandemic has yielded unique emotional blends and states of mind, many laced with anxiety. Most anything around us served as metaphor—a magnolia bush, a cat catching a mouse. A simple drive around a familiar but empty hometown felt disconcerting. Memories of old traumas resurrected themselves to help or hinder. Sleep cycles were disturbed. COVID-19 even caused a unique kind of strange dreaming.

VOICES
FROM AN
EPICENTER
Page 223

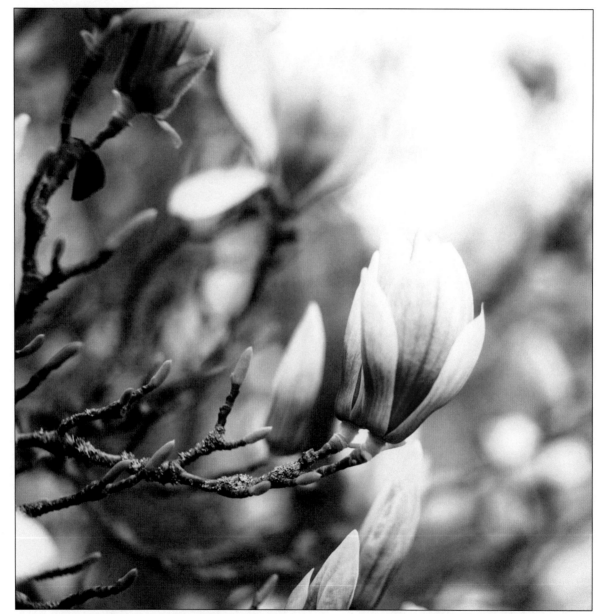

Spring magnolias (Photo by Marcus Spiske on UnSplash)

2020-05-16

Abigail Thomas

In spite of all that might be said, and despite what I have to say about all that might be said, today is sunny, and it's the sixteenth of May, the first day I don't need a sweater, and I'm sitting on the porch just sinking into spring. If I had a shred of ambition, I'd try to write a poem because I'm watching the ingredients of a haiku taking place right there in my yard.

My magnolia bloomed this year with such an extravagant display of pink and white that for weeks she has been practically afloat, putting words like wedding into my mouth, and bride, and I can't help staring because the wind, the errant wind is right this minute undressing my magnolia. Hundreds of loosening blossoms fall to the ground, and here come the adjectives, one after another—unruly, careless, impertinent, but I don't think she minds. She was probably getting ready to do it herself.

Forget the haiku. There are far too many syllables (luscious, deshabille, honeymoon) and here I am, left with only a title, *in flagrante delicto.*

Abigail Thomas has published two collections of short stories and a novel as well as three works of nonfiction: *Safekeeping, A Three Dog Life,* and *What Comes Next and How To Like It.* She lives in Woodstock, New York with her dogs.

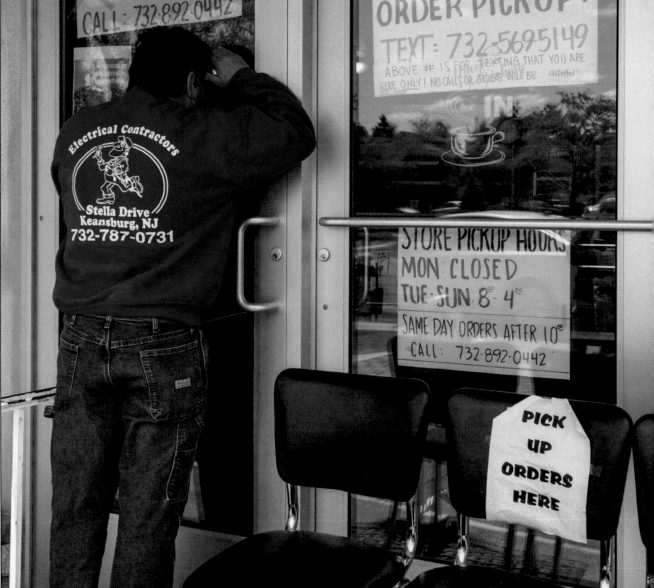

Whatcha Got?
An inquisitive man peers into a popular Jersey Shore bakery, May 7, 2020 (Photo by Jessica Margo)

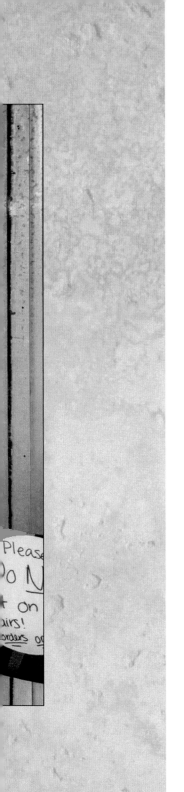

The Decision

MaryLynn Schiavi

June 27, 2020

His little mouse face contorted in agony as I moved him from my kitchen to the backyard. He was the victim of the little tiger, my cat, who sleeps by day and roams the jungle of my home by night. With his legs mangled, half torn away, he would never walk again. Clearly, he was in pain and now he was suddenly under my care—a job for which I never applied.

My breathing became heavy. *What choices do I have?*

My thoughts turned to health-care workers on the front lines of COVID-19, helping those whose respiratory systems were mutilated by this virus and for whom death was inevitable. *How do they help ease their patients into death?*

My thoughts wandered back even further to my mother's last day in the hospital. The doctors said there'd be no way she could breathe on her own. Suddenly it was my responsibility to decide how to ease her into death.

These months under quarantine, my thoughts have traveled back and forth from that hazy corridor leading to death. *Will this be my time? Or will this virus yank those I love from my life?* And at what point do we give up and turn to the agonizing question of how to ease into death?

In my yard the question was before me again: what choice do I make for this living being wrapped in pain, with no hope of survival?

A friend suggested unleashing the tiger who began the malicious deed or a swift blow to the head. Both options were out of the question. I could have simply left him in the woods to pass away slowly on this ninety-degree day, but that, too, seemed cruel.

My thoughts turned to my mother again, many years earlier: the morphine was administered, her lungs slowly shut down, and she closed her eyes for the last time.

Lacking morphine, I placed him in a plastic bag, helping to slow and cease his respiration, and lowered him into the earth. I quickly covered his tiny grave with dirt.

Still, I am haunted with questions, as many doctors and nurses must be: Did I make the right choice? Did I do everything I could have done? Was there a better alternative?

Why was I presented with this choice?

Where are they now? Do they blame me or thank me for easing them into death?

Do we even have a right to end someone's pain?

There are only questions, no good answers.

May they all rest in peace. May he rest in peace—for I surely won't.

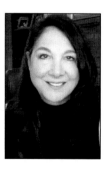

MaryLynn Schiavi is executive producer of Prosperity Communications LLC and *The Secret Flight,* a feature film and series. She lives in New Jersey. Twitter @MaryLynnSchiavi; www.prosperitycommunications.net

CORONA
CITY
Page 230

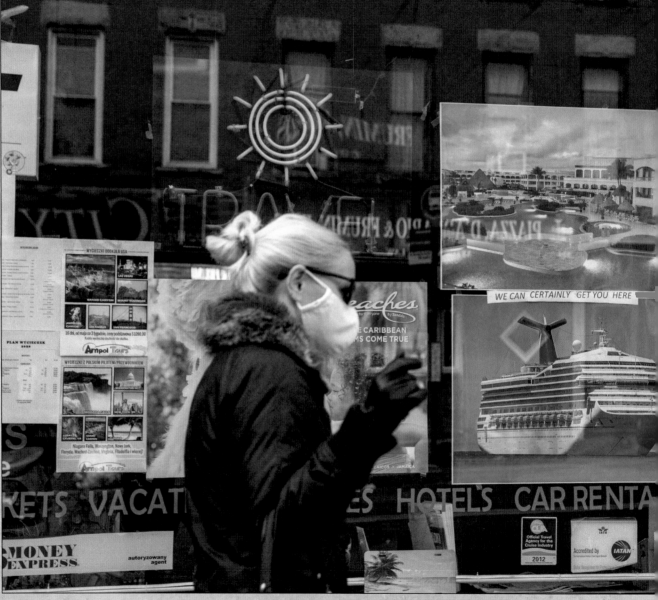

Impossible Dreams
Greenpoint, April 12, 2020 (Photo by Walter Wlodarczyk)

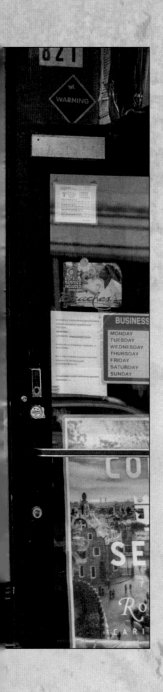

6:20 a.m.

Kathleen Cronin

April 13, 2020

It's 6:20 in the morning and I can't sleep. I woke up at 4 a.m., my chest feeling heavy. I'm worried. *Do I have COVID-19?* I've had some mucus and, now, a slight headache.

Weeks ago I found two unused N95 masks in the closet among the paint cans. Painters I'd hired several years ago had left them behind. They're still in good condition. Finding them brings a welcome relief. But if I wear one outside my house, will I be scorned, even condemned? Hospitals are so short of supplies.

Yes, I donned my N95 the other day and went to Rite Aid for a Brita water filter. I filled up the cart. Customers walked up and down the narrow aisles, all without masks. When someone came into my line of vision, I veered in another direction or at least made the attempt.

Yesterday I went to Rite Aid again, that time wearing a homemade mask. It didn't fit tightly around my mouth and nose. Much to my relief, though, every shopper wore a mask. My cart was full again when a very large man stood next to it in the frozen section. I blame myself. My cart was in his way. I immediately moved it as he stood there, singing aloud, nonstop. He kept singing as he walked throughout the store. To hear him both amused and terrified me. How is it that a jolly person terrifies me? Germs. Fear. COVID-19 spreads in the air and the volume of airborne droplets released by singing is six times more than those released by talking.

Oh yes, I almost forgot: I had a doctor's visit Friday—four days ago. I'd had an irritation at the corner of my right eye. I drove to Paramus with my trusty N95 mask and parked in the doctor's driveway. Following instructions, I called to let the staff know I was there. Someone came out and escorted me into the office. No other patients were allowed while I was there. A yellow and black caution banner was taped across the front of the receptionist area. Everyone on staff wore a mask with one exception—the receptionist. Why not the receptionist?

The rain is coming down hard today. It is not letting up, like the pouring in of uneasy feelings. Fearing the beast, I won't venture to the store again. The heaviness in my chest from 4 a.m. is still with me. And it's still mixed with anxiety—not a good combination. I drink a variety of hot teas and take probiotics as well as numerous vitamins, including high doses of vitamin C and doctor-formulated Deep Immune Health. All this in the hope my immune system will be so strong, no virus can penetrate it.

I just listened to Chris Cuomo's short video on how he is overcoming COVID-19. Don't become sedentary, he says. Don't give up your strength to the virus. Keep moving and fight back. That's a motto I adhere to, even on four-and-a-half hours of sleep. I'll be exercising at home. There are plenty of online classes. Thank goodness for Zoom.

Each country has had its own way of dealing with COVID-19. New Zealand's prime minister acted quickly. Only five deaths have been reported there. Her response saved and protected New Zealanders, whose government also will provide for them financially. The polar opposite is true in the US, though. Here deaths are in the tens of thousands. Our situation is sad and, more than that, petrifyingly tragic.

I've done my share of crying but I must not give in to the pain, both emotional and physical. I will continue my religious practice, praying and chanting for those who don't have the strength to do so for themselves. And after that I will take a walk, connect with loved ones by phone, take pictures of my garden, and post them on Facebook—all an effort to keep my mind and body healthy.

I long for the day we can meet each other on the other side of this devastating storm. The sun will come out again on some unknown tomorrow but, sadly, not for everyone.

Kathleen Cronin taught elementary education for the first sixteen years of her career in the New Jersey public schools. For the past seven years she has been a learning disabilities teacher consultant. A lover of cultural and creative arts, she is currently working on a novel and a memoir.

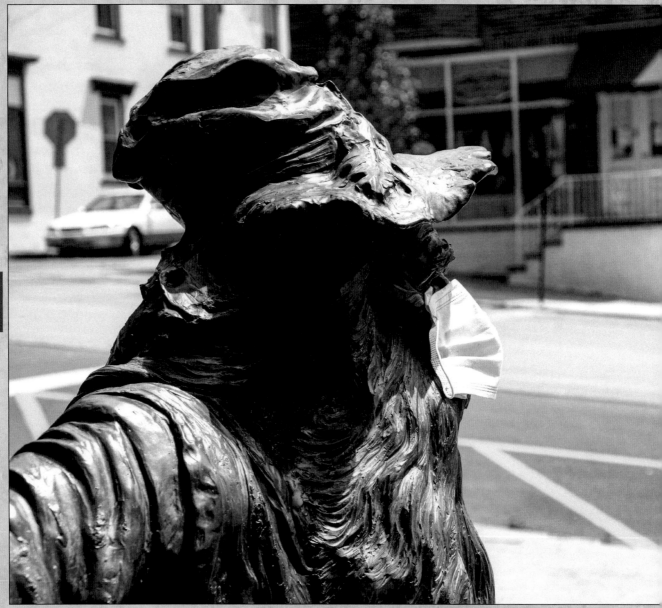

Masked Rip Van Winkle
A life-size bronze Rip Van Winkle statue in Irvington, New York, wears a
mask during COVID-19 lockdown, May 15, 2020 (Photo by Arielle Young)

In My Dream

Leisha Douglas

There were only machines, pills and vaccines,
no more nurses, no more doctors.
Restaurants where people sat and waiters hovered,
gone.
Gone too, spas and salons,
all promises of rejuvenation and care.
The only open bars, twilight dark,
furtive patrons in opposite corners.
Parties, weddings, funerals,
bracketed faces attending by computer.
Trains and planes in motion but almost empty,
movie theaters, concert halls, mostly relics.
People briefly formed small anxious clusters
then dissipated.
Smiles masked, hugs, handholds forbidden,
everyone dangerous.
The sun brazen in the clarified sky.
A flood of songbirds.
I wanted to wake up but couldn't.

As a psychotherapist for more than thirty years, Leisha Douglas enjoys her work, especially since it affords her the time to pursue her writing addiction. Her poetry and short stories have appeared in the *Alembic, Corium Magazine,* the *Cortland Review, HitchLit,* the *Minetta Review,* and *Upstreet* as well as other journals. She has been nominated for a Pushcart Prize in poetry.

CORONA
CITY
Page 236

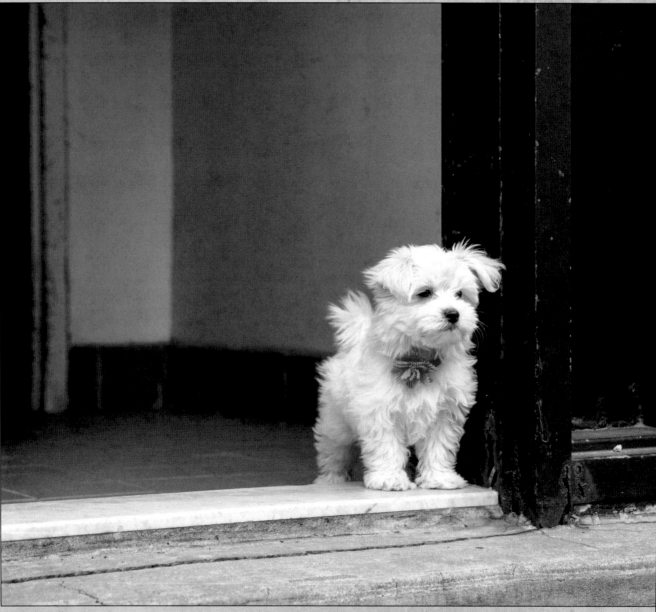

Corona Collar
Brooklyn, April 16, 2020 (Photo by Walter Wlodarczyk)

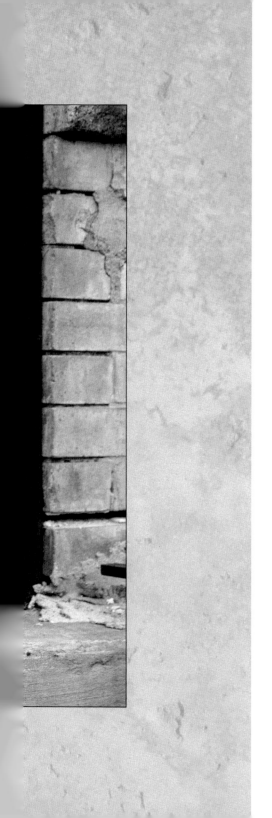

Spring Training

Ellen Bedrosian

March 31, 2020

Every year in late January, John, my best friend from college, dreams of Port St. Lucie, spring training, and the Mets. He prattles on about *this* player and *that* player and how happy he'll be watching America's pastime with reckless abandon.

Now it's spring and the only training in his life consists of sitting on the sofa, bathed in boredom and the washed-out hope of life ever returning to what it was— the everyday living we all took for granted.

Yet back in January (when pandemics were something that happened somewhere else in the world), while John anticipated the glory of spring training, I relished being here now in the damp and cold of a New York City winter. I thought about John as I practiced the gift of mindfulness meditation:

How silly it is to live for the future. A future that may never happen. There's so much to savor right now, right here. Icy winds freezing my nose as I walk crowded Manhattan sidewalks to see a Sunday matinee. Ice-coated tree branches sparkling like diamonds in afternoon sunshine. The fat, orange tabby purring on my lap. Even the dust bunnies lurking in the corners of my home bestow their own kind of joy. They let me know I have something to do. A chore. A purpose. And I'm still alive to vacuum.

In this time of the COVID-19 quarantine, spring baseball training morphed into mindfulness training for the masses.

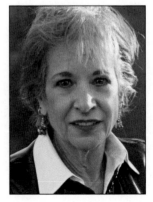

Ellen Bedrosian (aka E.B. Littlehill) is a writer and photographer who lives in Bergen County, NJ. She has published a chapbook of poems entitled *See the Dragons – A Collection of Zen Haiku* which explores three types of love: romantic, unrequited and spiritual. You can see more of her photos and writing on her website www.eblittlehill.com. IG: e.b.littlehill.

Self-Talk for Survival

Marcia Mickley

The internet showed constant coverage of COVID-19, of sickness and deaths. There were warnings that people over sixty were most at risk as were those with autoimmune disorders. Shocked, I realized I was at high risk.

My husband and I immediately cancelled all plans and appointments and socially isolated. The lessons I was taught as a child—that I was lazy, selfish, and couldn't do anything right—echoed in my brain. *I'm inept. How can I survive?* I became even more frightened.

Worries about having enough food and supplies caused stomachaches and then took over my thoughts. *How can I get fresh vegetables, toilet paper, and hand sanitizer?* Feelings of helplessness amplified and made me shake inside. Then the vivid flashbacks arrived and I relived the lack of safety and security I'd endured when I was young.

After three days of isolation, my fears froze my ability to think rationally. Realizing I had allowed desperation to grab control, I sat alone, snuggled deep in a plush, comfy chair, and closed my eyes. Years ago I'd learned that time and space away from my mother's insults and screams calmed me. *Would that work now?*

After breathing deeply in the quiet, the coping skills that I'd learned as the family scapegoat rushed back to help me. *I must make an immediate attitude change. I must adopt an attitude of gratitude.* Mentally, I listed all the ways I feel blessed, starting with my husband and children, the food on my table, and the roof over my head. I reminded myself that I'd already survived some very tough times and recalled when I was forced to leave home with only eleven dollars to my name. No, I was not helpless. I was resilient.

I told myself not to let fear overwhelm me and that, although I can't change the pandemic, I can change how I deal with it. Then I asked myself what skills I needed to be safe. An answer spilled into my mind: *This is the right time to grow a vegetable garden.* The need to be self-sufficient felt familiar. It had started when I was a child. I felt energized by the thought of growing food and finding new recipes. Here was an opportunity to develop new talents.

Still breathing deeply, I also felt sadness and a deep loneliness. *I can't expect much help from other people.* Then I turned that thought around: *I'm grateful I'm not in this alone.*

Looking to the future, I visualized a better time when the COVID sickness would be resolved and the world would be safe again. I envisioned my family staying healthy until that bright new day arrived.

Although I'd been taught that I was selfish, I ignored that lesson and donated one hundred fifty pounds of food to feed the hungry, called isolated seniors to ease their loneliness, and brought treats to my town's brave first responders to show appreciation for their efforts.

I hold tight to positive thoughts, but sometimes fear, frustration, and anger return. It distresses me when people refuse to wear masks, don't maintain a social distance, or heed recommendations to drink bleach. But I remind myself of another lesson I learned as an abused child: I can't control what others do. I'm responsible for my own choices and I choose to survive.

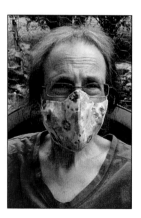

Marcia Mickley is writing a memoir about her journey from a childhood of abuse to an adulthood of serenity and healing. Her goal is to highlight resilience in life's darkest times.

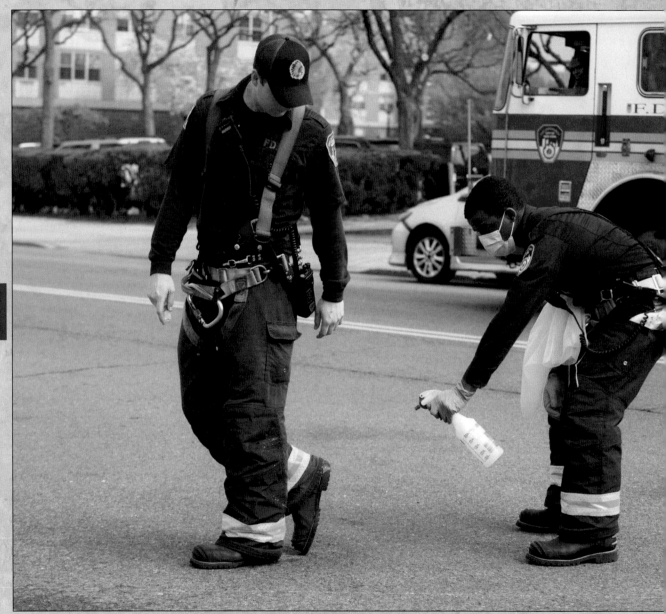

Can't Sanitize Enough
A New York City firefighter from Engine Company 257 in Brooklyn sprays down a colleague's boots
after they worked on a COVID-19 patient in a nursing home, April 15, 2020 (Photo by Lloyd Mitchell)

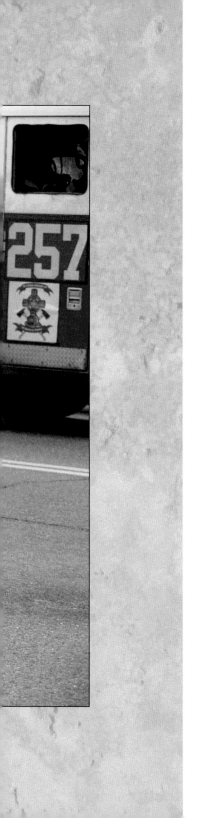

A Fierce Resilience

Liz O'Toole Papazian

June 17, 2020

When I first saw images of an empty Times Square and Broadway in the news, they frightened me. The reality in March 2020 was that the COVID-19 pandemic had exploded and finally reached the US. And my hometown, New York City, was in lockdown. People in hazmat suits were everywhere. Doctors, nurses, and EMTs wore them while treating those who'd contracted the virus. As an Irish American, I was stunned to learn that the Saint Patrick's Day parade was cancelled for the first time in 257 years.

After a few weeks, I ventured out of my safe suburban home to the supermarket, only to find entire aisles of paper goods and cleaning supplies empty. Each masked shopper was instructed to practice social distancing. At the checkout counters, plastic guards, hung like military shields, separated cashiers from customers. I felt fear in the air and saw it in people's eyes—a raw, lonely fear I've never before felt.

When driving, I read illuminated signs that read: "Stay home, be safe" and "We're NY tough." *Are they supposed to help me feel better?* Being New York tough exhausted me. Besides, news footage told a different story: Sick people were lined up outside city hospitals, waiting for treatment like weary soldiers. Refrigerated trailers on Randall's Island were being used as overflow morgues.

When I studied the flu pandemic of a hundred years ago, my fear of dying intensified. It killed almost 675,000 Americans—and fifty million people worldwide. *Will I or someone in my family or friends be one of the statistics this time?*

With nowhere to go, I felt anxious, frustrated, and overwhelmed. My hands became raw from washing so often. I slept more. I passed the time on house projects and Netflix. Our border terrier was happy with his extra walks, but we noticed he, too, was out of sorts.

Planning for college tuition and retirement amidst a wildly fluctuating stock market caused a panic I still can't put into words. Finally, I understood what my grandparents must have felt during their young lives in the Great Depression. My feelings spiraled from fear to anger to powerlessness.

Online meditation and writing groups saved my sanity. When I was finally able to put my terror in a little box in a safe corner of my mind, I clung desperately to the positives and reminded myself: *I'm able to work from home. My husband still has a job. My family is well.* On walks in the woods, I noticed green grasses and purple wildflowers appeared brighter. I observed a honey-colored deer creep through the brush and enormous, thick, old oak trees rise toward the sky, their canopied branches protecting me. Fresh air stroked my skin. At home food tasted sweeter and music sounded clearer. The truth was, even in a pandemic, I was blessed.

When I witnessed drive-by graduation celebrations, with horns honking and people cheering, my fear turned into confidence. In the same way, the family and friends of a woman celebrated her hundredth birthday. As she sat in her wheelchair, smiling and waving from the front lawn with creased hands, the look on her face quelled the shock of what we were living through, even if just for a few moments.

Even now as I watch the camaraderie of people in the tristate area, my pride is heightened as a native New Yorker, as it was during the 9/11 response. Restaurant owners and mothers donate food for frontline workers. Teens make masks. To me, the nightly clapping and cheering to support healthcare workers is nothing short of poetry in motion. All these acts reveal a fierce resilience.

As Governor Cuomo reopens the state now, the fear and anxiety I felt three months ago has subsided. I've learned a valuable lesson. I'll never question the good, the beauty, and the fragility of life again, even through the most daunting times.

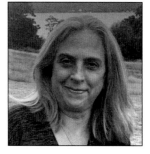

Liz O'Toole Papazian was raised in New York City and lives in the Hudson Valley with her family. Her work has appeared in the 2016 Brooklyn Film & Arts Festival, *RavensPerch, Pif Magazine,* and www.Boomercafe.com. She is currently polishing up her first novel.

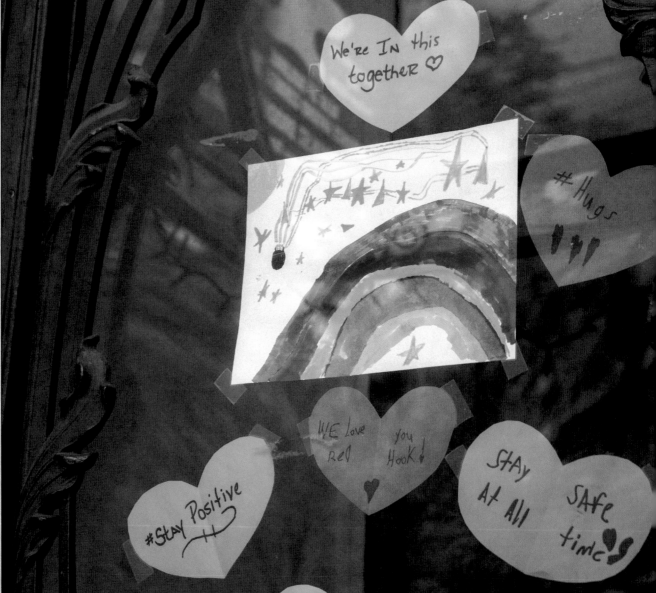

Children Are Our Future
Red Hook, April 16, 2020 (Photo by Walter Wlodarczyk)

FUTURE

So what's next? How do we live in stasis and plan for the future? What might the future look like, and when does it even start? We think about how the world may change and how we will change with it. Yet, even as we pine for our pre-pandemic lives, the opportunity to course-correct in a new normal excites us, too. We are human beings, which means hope springs eternal.

VOICES FROM AN EPICENTER Page 247

CORONA
CITY
Page 248

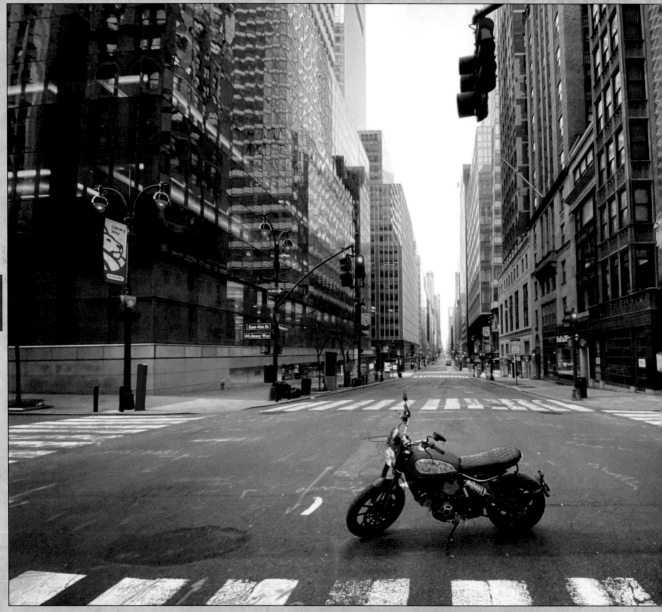

All the Right Traffic, All the Wrong Reasons
Madison Avenue looking toward Forty-Second Street during New York's citywide lockdown, with only a rebellious motorcycle breaking the grid, April 12, 2020 (Photo by Ethan Bregman)

Dreams on Hold

Ellen O'Neill

I'm Ellen, forty-nine years old. It's June 28, 1987. My husband gives me the best gift ever. He unlocks the door to 3 First Avenue, Apartment 12 and carries me over the threshold, saying, "I give you your dream."

There's the Empire State Building! I can see it clearly through the parlor window. This is a miracle. I'm starting a new life in The Big Apple. I'm going to live happily ever after. Thank you, Jim. You too, God.

■

Ellen here at sixty-three. It's September 11, 2001.

Oh what a beautiful morning! I'm beginning Austin Pendleton's scene study class today. Everyone who is anyone wants to take his class and he chose me!

In a rush to get to the bus I'm stopped by primary signs and brochures. *I'll vote later*, I think. *There's the bus.* As I step onto it, I catch God knows what exploding into a twin tower.

"Did you see that?" I yell. "What just happened?" A passenger calls back.

"Oh my God, the Pentagon is being attacked."

The bus reaches Fifth Avenue and the World Trade Center looks like a sun that's fallen aground. *Am I going to die?* I turn around. Everyone's terrified, just like me. I hear, "Abingdon Square, last stop."

The towers are gone. I wonder, *Is the class I was so looking forward to happening?* It is. It's full.

"You probably want to call home," Austin says. "There's a pay phone in the hall. One call each."

I dial my mom, who is eighty-two and teetering on the edge of dementia. I pray I can get my husband and children later. *Dear God, keep them safe.*

"Are you alright?" Mom cries.

"I'm fine, Mom. I love you." Austin dismisses us. "I'll see you next week." *Will there be a next week?*

With no trains or buses, I walk for miles. Running up First Avenue is a man wearing a jacket, shirt, and tie but no trousers.

"Give blood!" he screams.

I do not give blood. I visit mom. I don't vote. I go home and wait for hours for the phone to ring. It does not. I wait for my husband to come home. I wait. He arrives at 11 p.m. He's walked from the Bronx. He's okay, he's okay.

My kids finally get through.

"You can't live there anymore," they all say. "Come home, please."

No. I love New York. Of course I love my children, but I'll be damned if I'll let terrorists win. I'm living my dream.

■

Yeah, it's me, Ellen, still here at eighty-two, still here in New York City. Yes, I maintain my suburban home in Salt Point, too. And yes, I see my kids and my wonderful grandchildren all the time. I am living happily.

It's February 28, 2020. We've left a show on Forty-Second Street and are onto another. We stop for *halal*, picnic in the car, and munch chicken gyros between sips of white wine. At seven, we watch *Cambodian Rock Band.* The woman next to me is coughing up a storm. *Should I worry? Nah. The virus is in China, Italy, Washington.* I enjoy the show. Afterwards, I travel to my home upstate.

We are flying to Florida this week to celebrate my grandsons' eighteenth birthdays. Suddenly, Skype beeps and bubbles. I answer to my delights, Joseph and Michael. They are begging me.

"Oma, don't come," they say. "We're afraid for you. If anything happens to you, we'd die."

I can refuse my grandchildren nothing. After I spend two days on hold, JetBlue responds: we're cancelled. Since then I stay imprisoned in my log cabin. At first it's a relief to be stuck indoors. I clean drawers and closets. I take walks in the wild with deer, assorted crawly creatures, and wildflowers. There are no FDR Park joggers. No restaurants are open, so I cook all the recipes I've collected for years. I meditate via Zoom.

I am not alone. I can kiss my husband and he, me. That's good, but I miss touching and holding my family and friends. For the first time in my life, all the people dying in my country and the world are in my daily prayers.

I'm the same age as my mother was in 2001. Am I too old to adjust? Will I be alive when this is over? Will it ever be over?

I continue to clean. As I do, I surrender dreams. What about all those projects I intended to do? Should I throw them all out? I like donating to thrift shops. Will they even exist after coronavirus? And New York City, the city I love, must I give it up? Dear God, the questions are plaguing. How can all this death and all this change ever beget a happily ever after world?

And what does the future hold for my grandchildren? Dear God, what does it hold for *me?* Are there any dreams ahead? Dear God, Dear God.

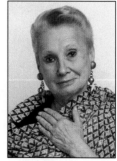

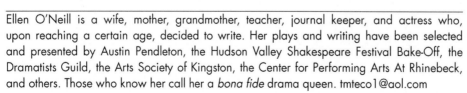

Ellen O'Neill is a wife, mother, grandmother, teacher, journal keeper, and actress who, upon reaching a certain age, decided to write. Her plays and writing have been selected and presented by Austin Pendleton, the Hudson Valley Shakespeare Festival Bake-Off, the Dramatists Guild, the Arts Society of Kingston, the Center for Performing Arts At Rhinebeck, and others. Those who know her call her a *bona fide* drama queen. tmteco1@aol.com

Caterpillar to Butterfly

Robert Cubby

June 30, 2020

At times the downtown area where I live appears to be a war zone. It's abandoned, shuttered. No one is out walking. Those people I see occasionally are wearing masks. They walk with their heads down, as if they're in some other world, far from the sight of all they've lost. It's an unemotional scene because masks hide our facial expressions. Indoors we all move in the same directions, following arrows on floors and signs on doors.

The far future—even the near future—is uncertain at best. The virus changes so rapidly. I'm still not sure what direction I'll take. All I know is that every activity I took up is now gone.

After my wife died three years ago, friends got me involved in lots of activities—senior gym class, senior trips with the local recreation department, the Senior Olympics, even Happy Hour at the St. Moritz Grill with seniors from all these groups. I went swimming at the YMCA, took dance classes, sang in my church choir, and performed in community theater.

As the death tolls have risen, all those activities died, too. I grieve the loss of those who've died and the life I'd rebuilt. Listening to projections, I suspect life as I knew it will not ever exist again.

I've been down this rocky road before. When I was diagnosed with a crippling leg injury and told I'd never walk again. When I was diagnosed with PTSD stemming from my service as a police officer. When my wife died. My life has been torn down and changed many times, just like a caterpillar changes into a butterfly. Yet, as with every butterfly, the change from a lower existence to a higher one was always magnificent, miraculous.

A caterpillar can't stay the way it is. Transformation is inevitable. I feel we're being asked to do the same in this pandemic. We cannot, ever, return to what we once were. It's too deadly. Too many people will die. Those now trying to hold onto the past are already dying.

So at this point I have to take inventory: what do I need in my cocoon before I emerge as a butterfly? First, masks are not optional. They are the new attire, so I might as well make them look good. I've ordered fashionable prints.

Social distancing will mean no hugs, handshakes, kisses, or embraces for the foreseeable future. That impacts my social group greatly. We are big huggers and kissers.

Wiping down surfaces, staying home if I feel ill, working from home as much as possible—these are all common-sense measures our mothers taught us as children.

Mass gatherings for graduations, weddings, and sporting events will have to change. Bigger and better stadiums will have to become safer and responsible. So will commuting on mass transit. As much as we want to pack ourselves in like sardines, we can't anymore.

We're now safely in our cocoons and feeling closed in, stifled. We want to break out because all this safe distancing is stifling. Some of us want to push for the next stage, ready or not. But we're simply not ready. We haven't sufficiently changed as a society, as a world population. We still have much to work on.

I can't say what the new butterfly will look like. No doubt it will be beautiful, full of new life, colorful as it flies on the gentle breezes of life. But we must fly together. We are no longer a group of individuals. We are a collective whole. When one suffers, we all suffer. And that includes the Earth herself.

The life of the new butterfly will not be based on being busy all the time. It won't go to work or school every day. I see lives lived partially at home, partially at the office or in the classroom. That means less traffic and less mass transit on any given day. Nature will be happy. She seems happy so far with our COVID response. Let's not blow it.

As we all emerge as butterflies, none of us will be crawling on our bellies for an existence. Everyone will fly equally high, full of life and color. I wish these lessons could have been taught without such loss of life. But there is only one way to go now—forward.

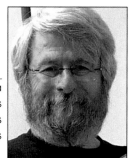

Robert Cubby, a retired police captain with the Jersey City Police Department, facilitates a support group for first responders and veterans diagnosed with PTSD. He also volunteers on several mental health boards in Sussex County, New Jersey, and assists senior citizens through the NORWESCAP Senior Help Line. A Reiki Level 2 practitioner, he interns in this Japanese healing art at The Tree of Health Center.

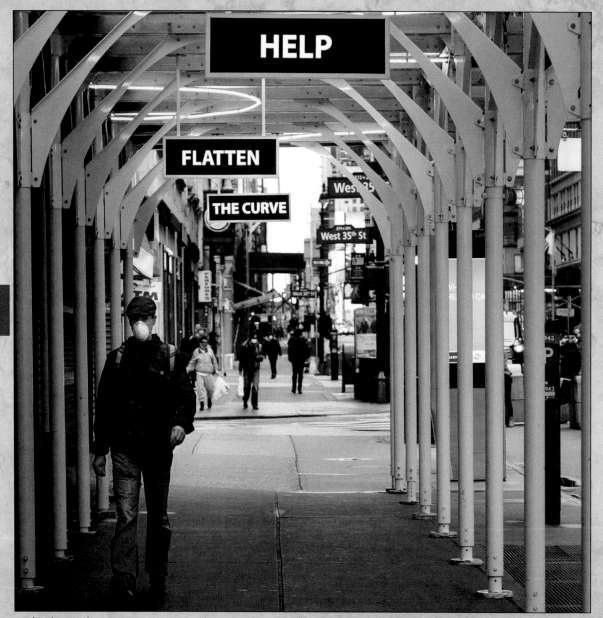

Help Flatten the Curve
Messages that encourage New Yorkers to do their part in the fight against COVID-19 pop up all around the city,
April 18, 2020 (Photo by Matthijs Noome)

Acknowledgments

Corona City: Voices from an Epicenter was conceived and executed as a charity project. Lorraine Ash Literary Enterprises, LLC, and Magic Dog Press, LLC, thank the following groups and individuals for their crucial help, freely and graciously given:

For hosting the first
***COVID-19 Diaries: Writing in the Age of Pandemic Zoom* series:**

The Mariandale Center: Karen Bernard and Jane Hanley

For lending their time and expertise, gratis:

Law Offices of Lloyd J. Jassin, New York, NY

Daniel Kulp, Asbury Park, NJ

Bill Ash Technical and Artistic Services, Allendale, NJ

Danielle Austen Photography and her "Photographer's Eye"
and "Photography Critiques" classes at the
Visual Arts Center of New Jersey, Summit, NJ

For our angel networkers and supporters:

Miriam Ascarelli
Laverne Bardy
Michelle Volle Borden
Janice Jencarelli Corrado
Beth Gershuny
Janina Hecht

Dan Hirshberg
Jason Ledder
MaryMichael Levitt
Colleen O'Dea
Jane Primerano
Mindy Reed at
AuthorsAssistant.com

Tehani Schneider
Lisa Vreeland
Barbara Williams
Maureen Wlodarczyk
Patricia Viscione Young

And especially, for heartfelt and artful work with their pens and cameras:
The Contributors

About the *Corona City* Team

Lorraine Ash (editor)

Lorraine Ash, MA, is a book editor, memoirist, and literary coach. A former journalist in her home state of New Jersey, she penned her first memoir, *Life Touches Life: A Mother's Story of Stillbirth and Healing* (NewSage Press), after her daughter, Victoria Helen, was stillborn in June 1999. Her midlife memoir, *Self and Soul: On Creating a Meaningful Life* (Cape House Books), followed in 2012. Lorraine believes in the power of first-person writing to bear witness, heal hearts, and change the world. She studied at Fordham University, Bronx, New York, and California State University, Long Beach. www.LorraineAsh.com

Sherry Wachter (designer)

Sherry Wachter, MA, started Magic Dog Press based on a single concept: stories need to be told. She and her business partner, Patrick Dunphy, provide professional and first-time authors a customized one-stop solution for getting books from concept to completion. They serve clients from coast to coast and abroad. Wachter's history spans book design, editing, and publishing as well as image restoration and illustration. She teaches writing and literature at Walla Walla University and Blue Mountain Community College in Oregon. www.magic-dog-press.com; www.magicdogpress.wordpress.com/custom-book-design

Dan Kulp (publicist)

Dan Kulp, BS, a marketing communications professional, has worked extensively in a variety of capacities in the lifestyle and consumer products industries. He develops innovative and persuasive media campaigns and marketing programs, online and offline, and enjoys strong relationships with influential media partners. Dan has served as vice president at lotus823 and RLA, both New Jersey public relations/marketing firms. He earned his advertising and marketing communications degree at the Fashion Institute of Technology in New York City. www.linkedin.com/in/dan-kulp

Lloyd Jassin, Esq. (lawyer)

Lloyd J. Jassin is a publishing and intellectual property attorney based in New York City and coauthor of *The Copyright Permission and Libel Handbook*. His practice includes drafting and negotiating licensing agreements, trademark search and prosecution, prepublication review of manuscripts for libel and privacy issues, and consulting on publishing matters. His clients include authors, agents, literary estates, publishing industry professionals, magazines, trade organizations, book and music publishers, and film and television producers. He also represents clients with intellectual property assets outside the worlds of publishing and entertainment. Before embarking on his law career, he was director of publicity for the Simon & Schuster General Reference Group. He earned his doctor of law degree from the Benjamin N. Cardozo School of Law in New York City and sits on the Trademarks and Unfair Competition Committee of the New York City Bar. He also serves on the advisory board of the Beacon Press, a nonprofit book publisher founded in 1854. www.copylaw.org

Bill Ash (proofreader)

In an interweaving counterpoint of arts and technology, Bill Ash has composed a career. Originally trained in architecture at Princeton University, Bill has also worked in computer support and training, technical writing and editing, website design and programming, book design and production, graphic design, and arts journalism. He now works in all these areas under the umbrella of his firm, Bill Ash Technical and Artistic Services. In concert with this he has enjoyed an active parallel career as a freelance musician, performing and touring in the New York area and around the country. He plays and teaches trumpet, trombone, and several other instruments. Bill also composes and arranges music. www.BillAsh.net

Photographers

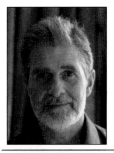

Tom Andrasz
Tom Andrasz is a practicing architect and amateur photographer residing in New Jersey. As an architect, Tom understands the importance of natural light and its interplay with and within the built environment. As a photographer, he understands the ephemeral nature of light, its ever-changing qualities, and its ability to evoke emotions and produce momentary works of art around us. Tom enjoys the creative process and draws inspiration from his surroundings. tjarchitect1831@gmail.com; Flickr @tja1831

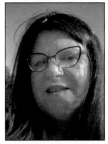

Lisa Bauso
Lisa Bauso is a photojournalist and lens-based artist. She is based in Brooklyn, New York and Portland, Oregon. lisabauso2@gmail.com

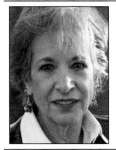

Ellen Bedrosian
Ellen Bedrosian (aka E.B. Littlehill) is a writer and photographer who lives in Bergen County, New Jersey. She has published a chapbook of poems entitled *See the Dragons – A Collection of Zen Haiku*, which explores three types of love—romantic, unrequited, and spiritual. www.eblittlehill.com; IG e.b.littlehill

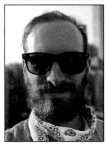

Ethan Bregman
Ethan Bregman designs racing engines for professional motorsport. His designs have been nominated for North American Race Engine of the Year. They've also won prestigious events, such as the Indianapolis 500, Daytona, the 24 Hours of Le Mans, and the FIA LMP2 World Championship. In his free time Ethan is passionate about motorcycles, architecture, and photography. ethan@ayton.nyc; IG ayton.nyc

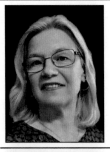

Charlene Federowicz

Charlene Federowicz of New Jersey graduated from the Rutgers University School of Communication and Information. After working in various industries, she now nears retirement and hopes to spend as much time as she can pursuing her passion for photography. She enjoys photographing nature as well as her grandchildren. cfederowicz@outlook.com

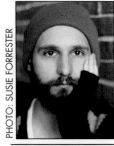

PHOTO: SUSIE FORRESTER

Daniel Freel

Daniel Freel most recently served as senior photographer at the *New Jersey Herald* from 2011 to 2020. During his tenure he received numerous New Jersey Press Association awards. His work documenting the pandemic was awarded second place in "Living and Photographing in the Time of COVID-19," an online juried showcase by The Photographer's Eye collective. Daniel has a BFA concentrating in fine art photography from Penn State University. freeldaniel@gmail.com; IG danielfreel; Twitter @freelphoto; FB Daniel Freel

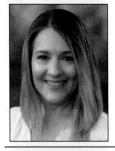

Jessica Margo

Jessica Margo of New Jersey graduated from the Center for the Media Arts, Germain School of Photography in Manhattan. She worked in a commercial still life studio and enjoyed a career in advertising and media. Her photos have been exhibited through the Visual Arts Center of New Jersey and at Studio Montclair. Recently Margo received four honorable mentions in the 15th Julia Margaret Cameron Awards, an international competition for women photographers. jessicamargophotography@gmail.com; IG jessicamargophotography

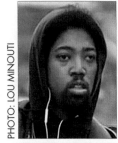

PHOTO: LOU MINOUTI

Lloyd Mitchell

Lloyd Mitchell, a photojournalist based out of Brooklyn, New York, has been photographing for the past eight years. He covers a variety of topics in Brooklyn for the *New York Times*, Reuters, *Canarsie Courier, amNY, Fire Engineering, Fire Rescue,* and the *New York Post.* lloydmitchellphoto@yahoo.com

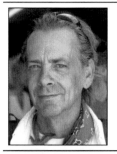

Christopher Monroe

Christopher Monroe has been a New Jersey-based photographer for more than thirty years. His work has been featured in various publications, including *National Geographic*, the *Record* and *Star-Ledger* newspapers, and *Automobile Magazine*.
chrismonroephoto@gmail.com; IG chrismonroephoto

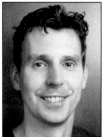

Matthijs Noome

Matthijs Noome is a self-taught photographer from the Netherlands who is based in New York City. As an avid outdoor enthusiast and nature lover, his main focus is nature and wildlife photography. He spends most of his free time capturing the urban wildlife of New York. Departing from his typical genre, Matthijs ventured out during the COVID-19 lockdown to document the city's empty streets, vacant landmarks, and drastically changed public life.
mfnoome@gmail.com

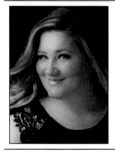

Rebecca Osso

Rebecca Osso is a photographer in Northern New Jersey specializing in family and event photography. She became interested in photography as a young teen and took her camera everywhere she went. Later, when her three children were small, she took night classes to perfect her skills. After the children grew older, she turned her passion into a business. Today she loves work more than ever.
rebeccaossophotography@gmail.com; www.rebeccaossophotography.com

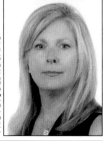

PHOTO: JOEL ROSANO

Diane Rosano

Diane Rosano started her career in print and TV journalism and has worked in the communications field, on and off, for years. A freelance writer, she recently launched SuburbanGrit, a feature magazine platform, on Instagram. She resides in Bergen County, New Jersey, with her husband, three kids, and two dogs. IG suburbangrit

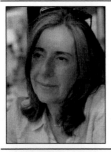

Emma Tager

Emma Tager, originally from Bogotá, Colombia, currently lives in New Jersey. Photography is one of her favorite pastimes. She is passionate about creating images both in urban and natural environments. emma.tager@gmail.com

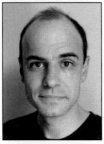

Walter Wlodarczyk

Walter Wlodarczyk is a documentary photographer whose work focuses on the stories and culture of his home, New York City. His photographs are a record of contemporary life in the city and a song to its continuous history of humanity and venture.
walter.wlodarczyk@gmail.com; www.walterwlodarczyk.com; IG wlodarczyk

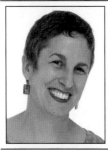

Joy Yagid

Joy Yagid is a New Jersey documentary photographer specializing in finding the intimate moments in life, big and small. Her work has been published in the *New York Times* and various local and regional online news outlets. Her nature photography has been shown in local, regional, and national exhibitions.
joy.yagid@gmail.com; www.joyyagid.com; IG joyyagid

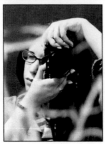

Arielle Young

Arielle Young of Elmsford, New York, graduated from Purchase College, State University of New York. During her sophomore year, while seeking a degree in journalism with a focus in Asian studies, she discovered her true passion for storytelling through photography. Inspired by outstanding professors, such as Nandita Raman, Robert Sabo, Donna Cornachio, and Renqiu Yu, she developed her street-photography style of covering journalistic events.
arielle.young@webleedshutterspeed.com; www.WeBleedShutterSpeed.com;
IG we_bleed_shutter_speed

Made in the USA
Coppell, TX
21 December 2020

46750863R00167